HEALTHY
HABITS

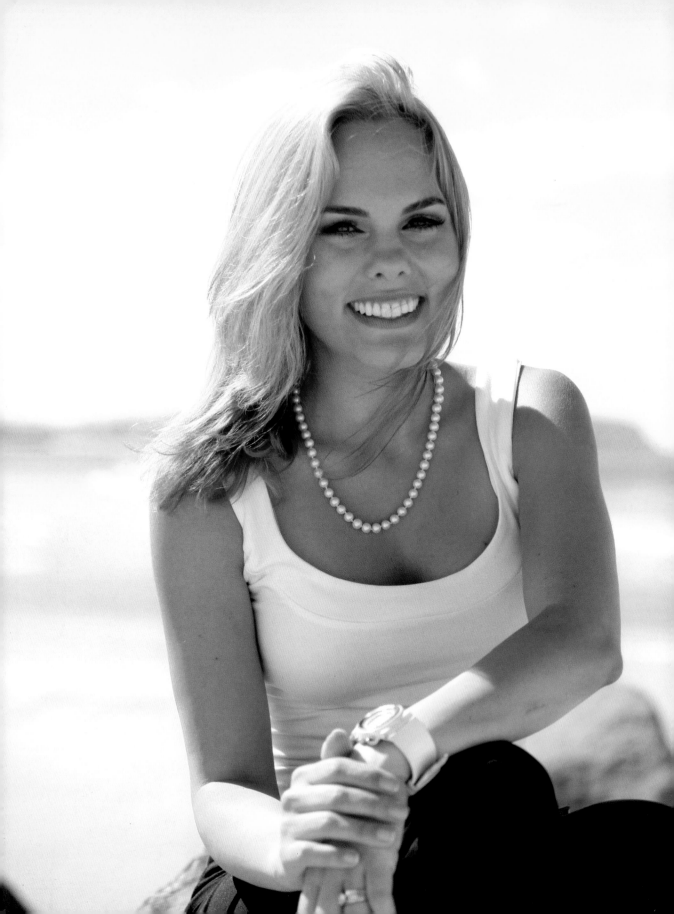

Healthy Living Series

HEALTHY HABITS

52 ways to better health

Dr CRIS BEER

ROCKPOOL
PUBLISHING

Healthy Habits – 52 Ways to Better Health is dedicated to all my patients and those I have had the privilege of helping over the years. You have all taught me so much! I have been humbled by your vulnerability to share your life experiences and challenges, and have been proud to share in your triumphs and joys.

A Rockpool book
PO Box 252
Summer Hill
NSW 2130
Australia

www.rockpoolpublishing.com.au
http://www.facebook.com/RockpoolPublishing

First published in 2015

National Library of Australia Cataloguing-in-Publication entry
Beer, Cris, author.
Healthy habits : 52 ways to better health / Dr Cris Beer.
9781925017540 (paperback)
Healthy living series.
Includes bibliographical references.
Food--Psychological aspects. Nutrition--Psychological aspects. Health behavior. Food habits.
152.33
Printed and bound in China
10 9 8 7 6 5 4 3 2 1

Cover and internal design by Stan Lamond
Editor: Katie Evans
Author Photographs by Bek Grace Photography
All other images from Shutterstock
Picture research by Andre Engracia

SOC Model on page 13 is used with kind permission from Prochaska and Diclementia Table on page 249 is used with kind permission from the Medical Journal of Australia conditional on all intended publications fully acknowledging the MJA as the original source of the content in the following manner: Samanek AJ, Croager EJ, et al. Estimates of beneficial and harmful sun exposure times during the year for major Australian population centres. Med J Aust 2006; 184(7):338-341. © Copyright 2006, *The Medical Journal of Australia* - adapted with permission. *The Medical Journal of Australia* does not accept responsibility for any errors in adaptation.

This book is for informational purposes only. Consult your health care practitioner for any medical advice. This book is not intended to diagnose, treat, cure or prevent a specific disease but offer geneeral advice only. The advice given in this book has not been evaluated by regulatory bodies.

Every effort has been made to locate the copyright holders of printed material. The publisher welcomes hearing from anyone in this regard.

contents

S i m p l e   H e a l t h   H a b i t s

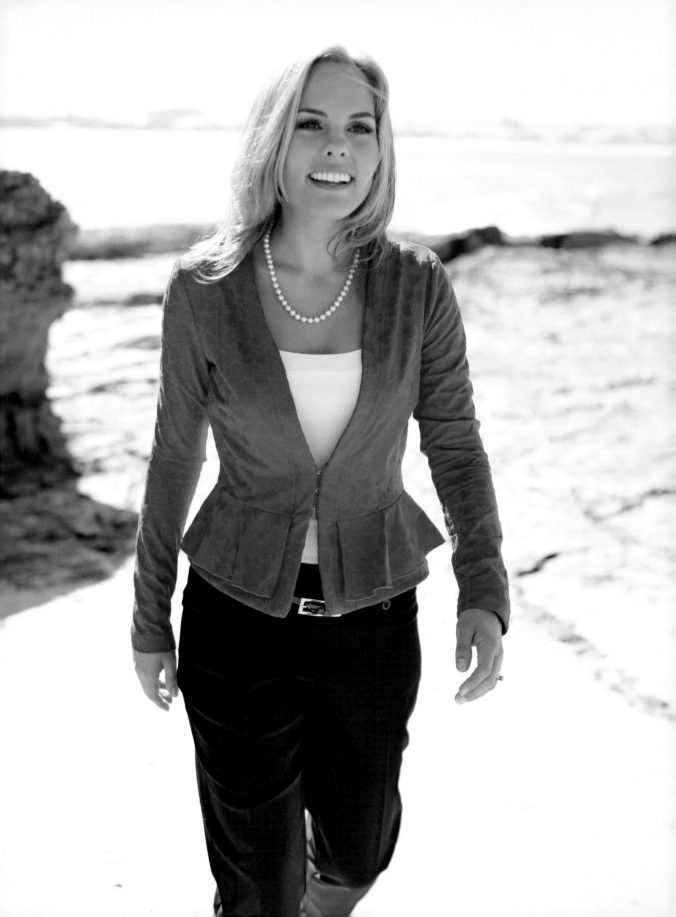

introduction

*Healing is a matter of time, but it is sometimes
also a matter of opportunity.*

Hippocrates 485 BCE

Have you ever longed to be healthy, have lots of energy, and be comfortable with your body weight? Well, then, this book is for you. *Healthy Habits* was written with you in mind and countless other individuals I have had the pleasure of professionally helping over the years. Their stories, perhaps much like yours, are marked by confusion and frustration at the myriad of conflicting health messages and advice available. None of which appear to be achievable in the busy lives that we all lead.

Healthy Habits is a book based on truthful and no-fuss health principles. This book is based on evidence and the principles should be easy to implement into our everyday lives. Although not appearing to be 'rocket science', when put into practice consistently true healing and health will be the result. After all, our bodies are remarkably complex but living healthily should not be. I have found quite the opposite. The simpler we keep things, the more likely we are to stick with any changes we make.

Aside from a professional call to write this book, I have a personal drive to write down what I have learnt from my studies as well as my experience. You see I too found myself in a place of frustration with my health in the early days of my career. Around 15 years ago I was diagnosed with high blood pressure and high cholesterol. After consulting a heart specialist it was suggested that I attempt to change my lifestyle or face having to take medication for the rest of my life in order to control my significant health risk factors. Feeling bewildered and terrified I decided to start learning all that I could about healthy living. This book is the culmination of many of the principles I have learnt through my studies in medicine, biomedical science, nutritional medicine, personal training and health coaching. It is also what I have found works with my patients as the principles are tried and tested many times over.

Healthy Habits offers a rare opportunity to discover all you need to know about how to be healthy, and have a waistline to match, in one book. By following the week-by-week advice within these pages you will see health emerge that you and your body deserve. You will start to regain the energy and vitality you thought you had lost, or had never previously attained. Your appetite and body weight will align with what is healthy for your frame. In essence, you will regain your health and, with it, your life.

your prescription

So how do you get the most out of *Healthy Habits*? Well, if you can humour me for a moment and allow me to use some 'doctor jargon', let me put it to you that this book is now your 'prescription'. It is your prescription to the great health, energy and waistline you have been searching for. If you follow this book like a prescription written from me, your doctor, to you, then those results will be your reality. But if you do not follow these tried and true principles, just like a prescription that is never filled, you will not achieve, or only partly achieve, the best results.

Healthy Habits is a week-by-week guide to improving all areas of your health including your mind, attitude and, of course, your body. You cannot separate, in my opinion, a healthy mind and attitude from a healthy body. They all go together. This book will essentially allow you to give yourself a check-up not just from the 'neck up', as the saying goes, but from the 'ground up'. There will be no part of you not overhauled in a positive way by *Healthy Habits*. Yes, fifty-two habits might seem like a lot but do not forget that you have a lifetime of habits to overcome and one year of your life to achieve great health is a short time in comparison to living a whole life not knowing what it is like to really feel and look good.

Consider perhaps taking a year to challenge yourself. Make this *your* year to really take control of your health again, or for the first time. Perhaps even ask a friend or loved one to join you in this challenge. This creates some camaraderie, perhaps some friendly competition, as well as, most importantly, some accountability. If you can be accountable to someone else you are less likely to give up because you do not want to let someone else down. Consider starting an online forum or blog to document your health changes. This is another way to create accountability.

As a way to visually record your progress consider using the week-by-week goal tracker labelled 'Your 52 Simple Habits Prescription' in Appendix A of this book. Tick off each habit as you work through *Healthy Habits* and as you start implementing those habits into your lifestyle. Remember to build on the habits from previous weeks by not neglecting those habits you have already established but add to them with additional positive habits. You may find some habits harder to implement than others. We will discuss more about why this might be in the next chapter on Habit Formation. You might also find you need more than just one week to implement a habit into your lifestyle. There is no problem with this, take as much time as you need. After all, life is a marathon not a sprint and just like a marathon you sometimes need to slow down to conserve your energy for the long journey ahead.

habit formation:
the key to getting & staying healthy is found in your habits

When was the last time you did something for the first time? According to Townsend and Bever[1], 'Most of the time, what we do is what we do *most* of the time.' That is, most of our behaviour is habit driven. We truly are creatures of habit. The good news is that if we can change our habits to be more positive we will find that our health drastically improves in turn. So what exactly is a habit?

What Is a Habit?

Habits are routine, usually unconscious behaviours performed on a regular basis. We start forming habits from birth. In fact, habits are adaptive behaviours, meaning they allow us to learn how to do something with the goal being to eventually be able to perform that behavior without having to think about it. A good example of this is driving a car. Initially, when we are learning to drive a car, we are very careful about every move we make. We may find that we are unable to concentrate on anything else except what gear to put the car in, or how far away we are from the car in front of us. But eventually, with practice, we no longer have to think about how to drive. In fact many of us probably drive to and from work and don't really remember the trip because we have engaged our subconscious mind to do the driving whilst our conscious mind is thinking about other things.

According to behavioural psychologists there are usually three components to a habit:

- **Repetitive** - meaning the action is something we do on a regular basis e.g. brushing our teeth before bed;

- **Automatic** - usually something we do without thinking too much about how or when we should do it e.g. driving a car; and

- **Situational** - situation-specific, meaning that we usually perform particular habits under particular circumstances e.g. eating snack food when watching TV (even though we might not be hungry, we are driven to eat in this situation).

So how exactly do we form a habit?

How Do I Form a Habit?

Habit formation is the process by which new behaviours become automatic. If you instinctively reach for a cigarette the moment you wake up in the morning, you have a habit. By the same token, if you feel inclined to lace up your running shoes and hit the streets as soon as you get home, you have acquired a habit. Old habits are hard to break and new habits are hard to form. That is because the behavioural patterns we repeat most often are literally etched into the neural pathways in our brains. Neural pathways are like highways - the more we repeat a habit the more 'worn' a highway becomes and the more difficult it is to break that habit. Changing our behaviour can be difficult and new behaviours might feel strange or unusual to us initially. This is because we are not used to doing them.

The good news is that through repetition it is possible to form positive new habits (and maintain them as well). This really is the key to creating a habit - practise it often. This starts the process of creating a new brain pathway. It takes around 21–40 days to form a new habit, so do not give up if the habit seems like hard work initially to maintain. Over time that habit will become an automatic behaviour and eventually a new lifestyle. This is the key to a healthier, happier you. You will be developing a lifestyle full of positive habits that will eventually be second nature and your new way of living.

A Word on Willpower

Willpower was never meant to sustain us. Consider willpower like the petrol in your tank. When you initially start on a long journey of change you may be determined to reach your destination. But as the journey progresses, you discover that the journey is actually a lot longer and sometimes a lot more uphill than you realised. Sooner or later you run out of petrol and have to stop. Sometimes we never return back to our journey of change to better health because the first time we tried it, it took too much effort. This is the problem with relying on willpower for long-term positive change.

The easier approach is to form good habits. Good habits are much like autopilot on a car. Once you have established them, which initially requires a short-term investment in energy and willpower, you do not have to concentrate so hard on the journey to good health. My advice is to stick with a habit until you have established it. Once this happens you move on to forming another positive habit in your life. Sooner or later you'll find you have established a whole new way of living; all without burning out in the meantime.

You may find you have developed a lifetime of bad habits by not exercising your will power in the short-term to redirect your behaviour towards choosing a more positive habit. So how do we break these bad habits in our lives?

How Do I Break Bad Habits?

Just like repeating a behaviour etches that behaviour into an established neural pathway, not practising a behaviour will start to cause that neural pathway to fade. It may never completely go away but it becomes less obvious. This means you are less likely to want to do that behaviour automatically. So to break a bad habit you first need to try and not do that behaviour at all (or as often). This involves removing yourself or avoiding a situation where you feel tempted to engage in that behaviour. If, for example, you find it impossible to avoid stopping at the local shop on the way home for a chocolate bar then one strategy might be to drive a different way home so that you are not tempted to stop.

Breaking bad habits also interestingly involves replacing them with better habits. If we simply aim to stop our bad habits and do not in their place add a better habit we will find we relapse. For example, if we stop spending our time in front of the television but do not find another enjoyable activity to replace the time spent watching TV then we will find ourselves tuning back in to our favourite shows.

Lastly, sometimes bad habits are filling a need of ours that is not being met. I have helped many people who eat emotionally because they are bored, lonely or feel unfulfilled. Seek to evaluate whether that bad habit is an attempt by our subconscious to meet a need, albeit in a not-so-productive way. Sometimes we need some professional help to break a habit. Consider speaking with your local doctor, counsellor or health coach if you feel this is the case.

So now on to some positive habits we can add to our lifestyles. These are laid out from habit 1 to 52, according to the weeks of the year, but are not in any particular order of importance. If you feel you have mastered some habits, gloss over these and focus on incorporating them into your lifestyle for 2-3 weeks before moving on to the next habit. At the end of each chapter is a breakout box titled 'Your Weekly Challenge'. This is what you need to actually do that week and can be easily referred to if you need to come back to a chapter later on.

know your motivators

When embarking on any change in your lifestyle it is helpful if you first identify what keeps you motivated. Everyone has different motivators for wanting to modify behaviours, and recognising what your reasons are will help to keep you focussed, especially when you face barriers or begin to feel resistant to change. The first part of this self-analysis process starts with defining what health means to you.

Health FACT

Only 50 per cent of people with chronic health conditions take the necessary steps to alter their lifestyle[1].

What Is Your Definition of Health?

No two people view health the same way. For some health might mean being free of aches and pains so that they can enjoy life to the full, for others it is about having enough energy to get through the day, and for others still it is about not dying young from something preventable. It is often useful to write your definition of health down and remember this when you are faced with having to make a decision about your behaviours.

Perhaps try finishing this sentence: 'Good health to me means …' (e.g. that I feel fit and am able to play with my children without feeling discomfort or pain).

Be careful not to write down specific weight goals as weight in itself does not determine good health, as explained in Simple Health Habit #21, which talks about being healthy at any size.

Strengthen Your 'Why?'

Once you have defined what good health means to you the next step is to strengthen your reasons for wanting to be healthy. These reasons will serve as powerful motivators for keeping you focussed. The stronger your 'why?' the stronger your resolve to stay the course to living a healthier lifestyle. Examples of what might constitute your top five reasons for why you wish to live a healthier lifestyle may include:

- To improve your energy levels so that you can fully enjoy travelling with your partner
- To improve your sex life
- To be able to enjoy exercise without experiencing pain
- To feel vital and youthful
- To be a positive role model to your children

Consider whether there have been reasons why you have continued with your current pattern of negative or not-so-beneficial health behaviours. In order to motivate you to shift what you are doing, your *reasons for wanting to change* need to be greater than your *reasons to stay the same*.

Along with defining 'health' and strengthening your underlying reasons for wanting to change it is also important to identify if you are truly ready for change.

Are You Really Ready?

Modifying any aspect of our health involves transitioning through what behavioural psychologists believe is six stages of change[2], as the schematic below indicates.

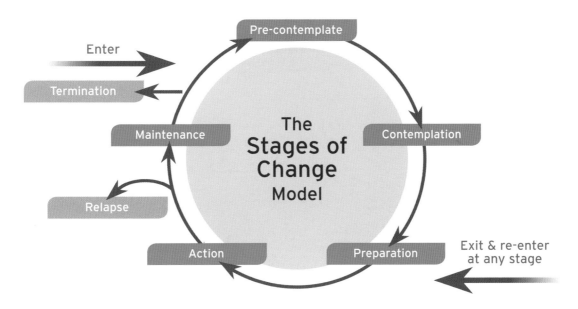

The first stage of change is where we **pre-contemplate** altering our behaviour. We may have thought about making some modifications to our lifestyle but have not made any specific plans to do so. It may not be the best time to change due to too many other distractions or disruptions in our life at that moment. If this is the case consider waiting until the dust settles a little and then re-evaluate whether you are ready. The next stage is where we have **contemplated** changing a little more seriously and may have started to gather information about what to do. This can often lead to determining that we want to change and being **prepared** to go for it. Following from this is deciding to take **action** and making specific plans and putting this into place. Along the way, once we have put in place some specific measures, we may find that we **relapse** back into our old behaviours. This is a normal part of the process and should not be considered a failure. Once we have established some new behaviours in place of old behaviours we have reached the **maintenance** stage of change, where these behaviours start to become our new normal.

By reading this book I am assuming that you are either in the **contemplation**, **action** or **determination** stage of change and are well on your way to making some positive new habits.

Rate Your Current Health

Once you have defined what health means to you, strengthened your reasons for wanting to make adjustments to your behaviours, and then identified where you are on the stage of change model and if it really is a good time to start changing, then you can rate where your health currently measures up. Consider the following six areas of your current health and rate each one from one to ten, with one being poor and ten being fantastic.

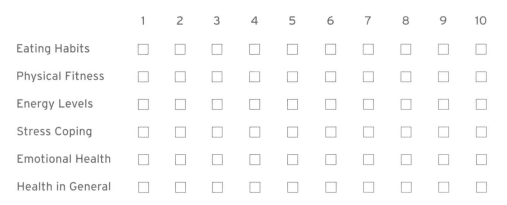

	1	2	3	4	5	6	7	8	9	10
Eating Habits	☐	☐	☐	☐	☐	☐	☐	☐	☐	☐
Physical Fitness	☐	☐	☐	☐	☐	☐	☐	☐	☐	☐
Energy Levels	☐	☐	☐	☐	☐	☐	☐	☐	☐	☐
Stress Coping	☐	☐	☐	☐	☐	☐	☐	☐	☐	☐
Emotional Health	☐	☐	☐	☐	☐	☐	☐	☐	☐	☐
Health in General	☐	☐	☐	☐	☐	☐	☐	☐	☐	☐

If you are not where you would like to be on the scale for each of these areas then consider what it would take for you to move up just one point. After all, it would be too much of an effort to move from, say, rating one to rating ten in one go. Small, progressive steps eventually get you there. An example might be if you are at rating five for energy levels, what would it take for you to get to rating six? It might be that you cut caffeine from 4 p.m. to avoid disrupting your sleep. Small changes make a big difference in determining whether we move up to the next level. Consider evaluating where you are on the scale once a month and writing down one or two things that you could try to help you move up one rating for each of the different areas of your health.

Know What Keeps You Motivated

Knowing what keeps you motivated will help you to stay focussed. Some people, for example, are motivated by rewards and others are motivated by recognition from others. If rewards are something that motivates you make sure you treat yourself after every achievement. Keep in mind that rewards, should be non-food based in order to avoid emotional eating. If recognition from others is your primary motivator then join a network where constant support will be available. Be careful, however, that you are not motivated to alter your behaviours in order to please someone else. Positively transforming your lifestyle should be about you and your health and not about appeasing someone else's wishes or desires.

What Is Holding You Back?

We all have reasons for why we may not have altered our behaviours already. We may have all the intentions in the world to change, but if there are obstacles preventing us then these need to be dealt with first before we can break free of negative habits. Some common obstacles include:

- Lack of time
- Lack of resources
- Lack of support
- Too busy at work
- Too many responsibilities
- Too tired or in too much pain
- Not knowing where to start
- Negative thinking

Identifying obstacles and then working to overcome them is a necessary step. There may be times where our responsibilities at work or home override our own needs. This is okay for a short period of time, but if we continue putting others first we will feel frustrated, resentful, worn out and eventually sick.

Identify Your Strengths

The next part of putting into practice positive health habits and overcoming barriers to change is to draw on your strengths. I meet so many patients, particularly women, who downplay their strengths and therefore feel powerless to make a start. Consider answering the following questions as a way to empower you to move forward in being able to make positive changes.

My strengths and what I have going for me include. (E.g. my ability to be organised and think rationally or my physical stamina.)

My strengths have assisted me in succeeding in an area of my life that required effort. (E.g. my ability to be organised means that I run a busy household whilst still holding down a part-time job; or, my physical stamina has helped me to keep going with long hours at work in order to meet a deadline.)

These same strengths can be harnessed and used in order to make positive changes to my health. (E.g. I can use my ability to be organised by working out a schedule that incorporates exercise and healthy meal planning; or, my physical stamina means that I can plan to exercise at the end of my day because I know I will still have enough energy.)

Be Prepared for Resistance

Any positive changes that we want to make in our lives *will* be met with resistance, so being prepared for this can help to keep you focussed. This resistance might be from external sources; for example, from friends who do not understand why you want to make healthy changes. This type of resistance is often a reflection of their own insecurities and guilt for not prioritising their own health.

The second type of resistance can come from ourselves in the form of excuses and self-sabotage. Making excuses is common and can be a normal part of change. Make a list ahead of time of the excuses you are likely to use, and come up with a list of reasons why those excuses will not hold. For example, an excuse might be that you cannot exercise because it is raining. An easy solution to this problem would be to have an indoor Pilates routine recorded or saved to your YouTube favourites.

Self-sabotage, on the other hand, tends to be more subconscious and can be related to feelings of low self-worth. If you find you always give up just when you are doing so well then this might be self-sabotage at work. If recognition of and steps to make adjustments to this behaviour do not work, then talking to a trained counsellor, psychologist and/or hypnotherapist might be necessary.

Make Your Plan

Once you have done the above exercises and identified your key motivators, strengths and barriers to change, it is then time to write down a plan for action. Use this book as a guide for areas you feel you need to work on. Write a very specific plan of the how, what, when, where and why for each of the areas you know you need to change. When you have mastered these areas then you can move on to others. Update your list regularly as you master new habits.

Take Home Points

In order to stay motivated when making positive health changes, define what good health really means to you.

- Identify your reasons for wanting to change. When the reasons to change are more compelling than the reasons for staying the same, you will find it easier to stay focussed.
- Recognise where you are on The Stages of Change model. This can help put some perspective on what to expect if you decide to embark on truly wanting to change.
- Rating current aspects of your health can provide an objective and measureable way to track your progress, which can help to keep you motivated.
- Many people find regular rewards and positive feedback from others two things that help to keep them motivated with making positive changes.
- Knowing what your strengths are and how you can apply these to the areas that you know need modifying is also an effective strategy for staying focussed.
- Be prepared to face obstacles and resistance to change. This is normal, and if you identify what these obstacles might be ahead of time, you will find the strength to overcome them.

YOUR *Weekly* CHALLENGE · · · · · · · · · · · · · · ·

This week your challenge is to identify your motivators, write down your strengths and your obstacles to change, and to make a specific plan to stay motivated. Use the exercises in this chapter as a guide on how to do this.

drink to good health

Water is the single most important nutrient that our bodies need and it is involved in almost every bodily function. With around 60 per cent of our body composed of water it is essential for life[1]. Even our bones are made up of about 30 per cent water[1].

Amazingly we can live for no more than 5 days without water as opposed to 30-40 days without food[2]. Yet many of us don't drink enough of this precious liquid. Most of us live in a state of mild to moderate dehydration and don't even realise it.

A recent patient of mine who is a plumber and works long hours outdoors was always suffering from muscle cramps and headaches. When I asked him how much water he drank per day he said the recommended 2-3 L. But when we undertook some general blood tests his results indicated that he was suffering from a state of dehydration with an alteration in his kidney function. I advised him to trial doubling his water intake. Within a matter of days his symptoms had improved. I recently saw him again and he mentioned that his symptoms have abated just by making sure he is drinking plenty of water to compensate his losses through sweat.

So what are some of the signs and symptoms that you may be suffering from dehydration? Some of these may surprise you!

Signs That You Are Dehydrated

- Fatigue[3]
- Headaches[3]
- Reduced concentration[4]
- Dark circles under the eyes[3]
- Muscle cramps[5]
- Dry skin[3]

- Joint pains[4]
- Dry, sticky mouth (late symptom)[3]
- Constipation[3]
- Dizziness or light-headedness[3]
- Inability to lose weight[4]
- Digestion problems[4]
- Decreased urine output (passing urine less than 4 times per day)[3]
- Dark-coloured urine[6]

Given these symptoms, how much water should we be drinking?

How Much Water Do You Need?

Although research isn't clear on exactly how much water to drink per day the general recommendation is 2-3 L per day or 6-8 glasses[6]. I generally make a more specific recommendation and say drink 1 L for every 25 kg that you weigh.

Keep in mind, however, that if you are engaging in heavy exercise or are sweating heavily then you need to add a extra 1-1.5 L for every hour of heavy exercise or heavy sweating[7].

You know that you have drunk enough water throughout the day if your urine is straw-coloured or clear.

Too Much of a Good Thing?

Sometimes when I am presenting a workshop on the importance of staying hydrated I am asked if it is possible to drink too much water. The answer is yes, you can have too much of a good thing.

There exists a psychological condition called psychogenic polydipsia where individuals are compelled to drink excessive amounts of water – sometimes reaching up to 20 L per day. At this level the body's electrolytes are diluted so much that there is a risk of seizures and brain swelling[7]. So you *can* drink too much water but, in reality, many of us are unable to drink the amount needed to be harmful. If you stick to the recommended quota you will be well within safe limits.

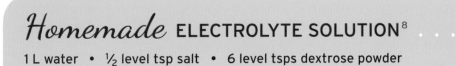

Homemade ELECTROLYTE SOLUTION[8] . . . .

1 L water • ½ level tsp salt • 6 level tsps dextrose powder

What About Electrolytes?

I am often asked whether it is important to supplement drinking water with electrolytes. The current research suggests that this is only important if you are undertaking heavy exercise for about 60 minutes or more or are sweating profusely[7]. In this case adding a few scoops of electrolyte solution to plain water is reasonable, or make your own by using the formula on page 19.

For the everyday individual who works indoors and undertakes light to moderate amounts of exercise plain water is the best option.

What If You Do Not Like Water?

Every now and then I meet individuals who do not like drinking water because they find it too bland. This is often the case if someone's taste buds are used to sweet or caffeinated drinks. As mentioned earlier in this book our bodies really only want what they are used to. If you are used to drinking anything but plain water that is what your body will crave.

As a personal example I remember a time when I used to drink diet cordial instead of water all day long. I was addicted to the taste and couldn't stand to drink plain water. When I came to the realisation that all that cordial was not good for my body and that I needed to switch to plain water I had a real mental challenge on my hands. I had to re-train my taste buds to crave plain water – which took me around a month to do. Now I can't imagine drinking anything other than plain water. My tastebuds have adjusted.

So what I say to individuals who are in the same situation is to keep at it. Continue drinking plain water until you are able to re-train your taste buds.

Some healthy additions to water are sparkling mineral water with lemon or lime juice or even some ginger and mint. On the topic of mineral water, some people find that they suffer from bloating and indigestion from drinking carbonated water – that is often because the water has been artificially carbonated rather than carbonated via a natural process. In this case try drinking naturally carbonated water such as Vittoria or San Pellegrino.

To Filter or Not to Filter?

To date there is no absolute evidence pointing to the benefits of filtered or bottled water over tap water in developed countries. Saying that, there is some preliminary evidence to suggest that the amount of chlorine and fluoride added to our water-purifying systems is harmful to our health and can be attributing to a number of health problems ranging from cancer and allergies to abdominal pains and headaches[4].

Tank water is prone to being contaminated with bacteria and other organisms[9]. I recall a patient who came to see me to seek help for abdominal pains and diarrhoea of three months duration. When we undertook stool testing she in fact had a parasite infection called cryptosporidium from drinking contaminated water. Tank water must be regularly checked to ensure it is not contaminated.

If you want to ensure that the water you are drinking is uncontaminated the best filtration system is reverse osmosis[4]. Make sure you purchase this from a reputable source. Many people choose to have a reverse osmosis filtration system installed under the sink. There is some evidence to suggest that choosing to add an alkaline filter to your system replenishes essential minerals in the body[4]. As an alternative to alkaline filters you can add a few drops of alkaline solution to each glass of water. Alkaline solution can be bought from most health food stores. Often bottled water is actually tap water filtered in this way and not 'bottled at the source' as marketing would have you believe.

Chilled, Warm or Room Temperature?

This is another common query. Should our water be drunk at room temperature, slightly warmed or drunk cold? The theory behind drinking warm water or room temperature over chilled is that chilled water is too much of a 'shock' to our body, which typically sits at around 37 degrees. To date, however, there is no supporting evidence to suggest warm is better than chilled. In reality, most of us are able to drink more water if it is at room temperature simply because chilled water is often too cold to drink at once.

Should You Wait Until You Are Thirsty?

By the time we actually feel thirsty we are already dehydrated. This is due to the delay in response from brain osmoreceptors - an area of brain tissue that literally detects when we are running low on water. The best approach is to be proactive about drinking water and to drink it regularly throughout the day.

Drinking your entire water intake at the end of the day because you have realised you haven't drunk enough unfortunately won't be of much benefit. This is because the body filters water at a certain rate, leading you to pass the excess water as urine. Waiting till the end of the day will most likely lead to disturbed sleep when you have to keep getting up to go to the bathroom! A better approach is to pace yourself and drink a glass or about 200 mL every 1.5-2 hours. If you find that you have to go to the bathroom more than once throughout the night try limiting fluids three hours before bed.

Lastly, an interesting phenomenon occurs when we become dehydrated. Our body confuses thirst with hunger. So the next time you are feeling hungry try drinking a glass of water to see if your appetite can be curbed.

Strategies to Increase Your Water Intake

Some ways to ensure adequate water intake are:

- Take a large 1 L water bottle to work and ensure you refill it at least once.
- Keep a jug of water on your desk and drink a glass every 1.5-2 hours.
- Choose water over juice or soft drinks at lunch.
- Choose sparkling mineral water at restaurants rather than another glass of wine.
- Add a little lemon/lime juice and mint to water for flavour.

Take Home Points

You need water to survive and thrive.

- You need on average 2-3 L of water a day or about 1 L for every 25 kg that we weigh.
- You know you have drunk enough when your urine is straw-coloured or clear.
- Dehydration can occur even when you are not thirsty. The most common signs and symptoms are fatigue, headaches, muscle cramps, constipation and light-headedness.
- Only add electrolytes to your water if you are undertaking heavy exercise for at least an hour.
- Our body tends to want what we normally give it. Over time, with consistent water drinking, our bodies will learn to love this vital liquid.
- If you choose to filter your water the best water filtration system is reverse osmosis with or without an alkaline filter.
- You can often drink more water if it is at room temperature.
- Try to drink consistently throughout the day by always keeping a bottle or jug filled with water near by.

YOUR *Weekly* CHALLENGE . . . .

This week your challenge is to increase your water consumption to 6-8 glasses a day or 2-3 L. If you are not used to drinking this much water, start by adding one extra glass a day until you build up to the recommended amount. Remember to spread out your water drinking throughout the day.

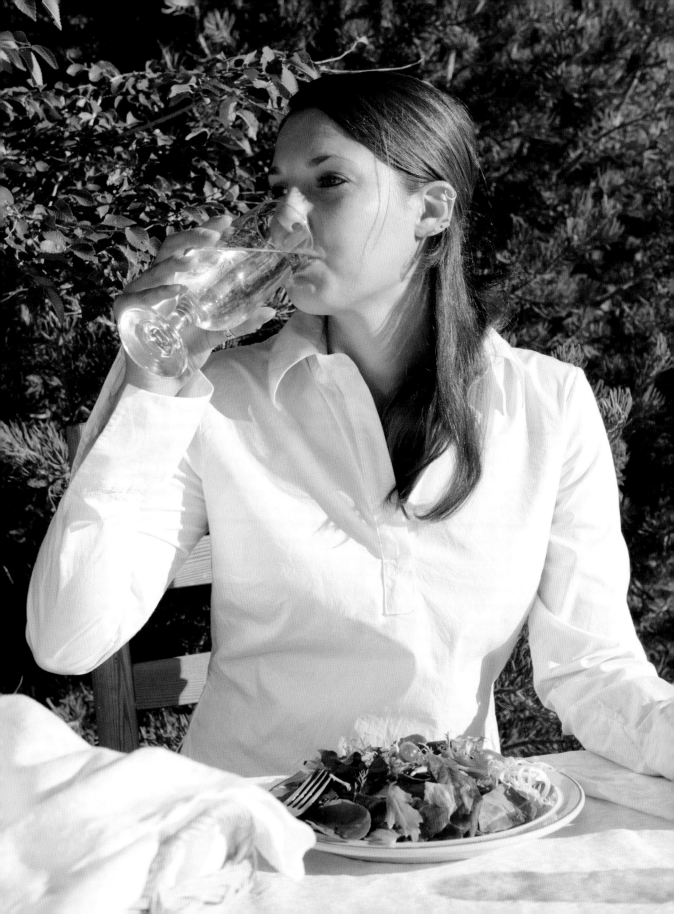

avoid shrinking your brain

As mentioned in the last chapter on drinking to good health, water is the single most important nutrient our bodies need. Hydrating our brain is especially important as it is composed of around 75 per cent water[1]. When we do not drink enough water our brain cells become dehydrated. This can lead to various symptoms ranging from mild to debilitating. I call these symptoms warning signs that your brain is 'shrinking'.

So what are some symptoms of brain shrinkage?

Common Symptoms of Brain Shrinkage From Dehydration

Dehydration of brain cells leads to the following symptoms:

- Headaches[2] (particular worse with movement, bending down or climbing stairs)
- Fatigue[2]
- Dizziness[2]
- Confusion[3]
- Reduced concentration and cognition[3]

What Does It Take to Shrink Your Brain?

A team of scientists in the UK found that 90 minutes of sweating without replenishing lost fluids shrinks the brain as much as a year of ageing[4].

The same study revealed that dehydration not only affects the size of the brain but how effectively it works. At just 1 per cent dehydration researchers observed increased brain effort required when performing common cognitive tasks such as short-term and long-term memory recall, maths calculations and general problem solving[4].

The good news is that the shrinkage and adverse effects on brain function can be easily reversed by rehydrating with adequate amounts of fluid. How to rehydrate is explained in detail in the previous chapter.

Aside from not drinking enough water, increasing the rate at which your body loses water through urine is a common cause of brain shrinkage. This is what happens when we drink alcohol and caffeine.

Caffeine & Your Brain Shrinkage

Caffeine is the most common drug consumed in the Western world[5]. It is a known stimulant and can be consumed safely in the right amounts.

The most common sources of caffeine include coffee beans, tea leaves, cocoa beans, kola nuts and guarana plants[6]. Caffeine can also be produced synthetically and subsequently added to various foods and beverages including tea, coffee, cola, chocolate, energy drinks and iced coffee.

A side effect of caffeine is that it acts as a diuretic by telling your kidneys to excrete more water. The more caffeine you drink, the greater the effect on the kidneys. This can quite quickly lead to dehydration especially if you are not drinking enough water to compensate.

It can be hard to know how much caffeine is in our food, so here is a table outlining common food and drink sources containing caffeine[6].

FOOD OR DRINK	CAFFEINE CONTENT	SERVE
Instant Coffee	60-80 mg	250 mL cup
Café Coffee (e.g. latte or cappuccino)	113-282 mg	250 mL cup
Espresso/short black	107 mg (25-214 mg)	1 shot
Energy drink	80 mg	250 mL can
Cola	36-48 mg	375 mL can
Iced Coffee	30-200 mg	500 mL bottle
Starbucks Breakfast Blend (brewed coffee}	415 mg 9300-564 mg)	600 mL ('Venti')
Black Tea	25-110 mg	250 mL cup
Green Tea	30-50 mg	250 mL cup
Milk Chocolate	20 mg	100 g bar

Sources: Food standards Australia New Zealand: Australian Institute of Sport Caffeine Fact Sheet

The safe amount of daily caffeine is around 200 mg for adults, 90 mg for teenagers, and very little for children[6].

Health TIP . . . .

The safe amount of caffeine for adults is 200 mg, which is equivalent to about 2-3 cups of coffee or 3-4 cups of tea per day.

Due to the fact that caffeine can be hidden in food products, especially those promoting improved 'energy' or 'weight loss', it is important to read the labels.

I recall one patient of mine who was having difficulty with insomnia, headaches and anxiety. When I asked her how much caffeine she had in a day she said that she thought she was having very little. But when we examined exactly how much she was consuming it was way above healthy limits. She was drinking on average 3 cups of coffee a day, one of these was a medium-sized latte from the local café, as well as 2 cups of green tea. She was also having a small chocolate bar for afternoon tea. This conservatively equated to a total of 350 mg of caffeine a day. In addition to the excessive amount of caffeine consumed, when we undertook some metabolic testing she was actually metabolising caffeine at a slow rate, meaning that it took her body at least 12 hours to clear 100 mg of caffeine (the average person takes 3-6 hours to clear this amount). No wonder she was having so many caffeine-related symptoms. When we reduced the amount of caffeine she was consuming her symptoms largely resolved within a week.

Another 'liquid brain shrinker' is alcohol.

Alcohol & Your Brain Shrinkage

Alcohol is a diuretic in the same way that caffeine is and therefore leads to dehydration in much the same way as caffeine does. Dehydration of the brain is the basis of a hangover. The more dehydrated your brain, the worse your hangover will be. To avoid a hangover try to drink a glass of water between alcoholic drinks.

Further to dehydration of the brain leading to brain shrinkage, the toxic effects of alcohol on the central nervous system have been shown to decrease brain volume over time.

As shown in the diagram on page 27 the areas particularly damaged as a result of alcohol are the[7]:

- **Cerebellum** - the cerebellum is the part of the brain responsible for muscle coordination. Damage results in difficulties with balance and walking, which is called 'ataxia'.

- **Frontal lobe** - the brain's frontal lobes are involved in abstract thinking, planning, problem solving and emotion. Damage results in cognitive difficulties.

- **Temporal lobe** – damage to the temporal lobe results in a loss of short-term memory, an inability to acquire new information and 'confabulation' (the person fills in gaps in their memory with fabrications that they believe to be true).

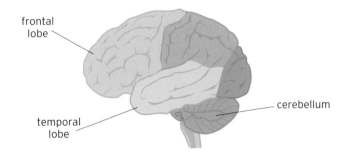

frontal lobe

cerebellum

temporal lobe

Health TIP . . . .

The safe amount of alcohol for an adult is no more than 2 standard drinks per day on 5 days of the week with 2 alcohol-free days per week.

The toxic effects of alcohol on the brain are most marked when you do not stick to the safe recommended alcohol limits. The current accepted safe alcohol drinking limits are[8]:

- For healthy men and women, drink no more than 2 standard drinks on any day.
- Try to have at least 2 alcohol-free days a week, preferably consecutive days.
- Drink no more than 4 standard drinks on a single occasion.
- No amount of alcohol is safe for those under the age of 17 years.
- No amount of alcohol is safe for pregnant women.

It can be quite a surprise to realise how much alcohol makes up a standard drink. Many people drink excessive amounts of alcohol without realising it. One standard drink is found in[8]:

- 100 mL of wine (red or white) – $\frac{1}{2}$ a wine glass
- 100 mL of champagne – $\frac{2}{3}$ of a champagne glass
- 30 mL of spirits or a 'nip' – $\frac{1}{4}$ of a spirit glass
- 375 mL of mid-strength beer – the amount found in a small bottle or can

Keep in mind that there are around 7.5–8 standard drinks in a bottle of red or white wine, 7.5 standard drinks in a bottle of champagne, 22 standard drinks in a bottle of spirits and 24 standard drinks in a slab of mid-strength beer.

Take Home Points

Our brain is composed of around 75 per cent water and is therefore very prone to dehydration.

- Symptoms of brain dehydration or 'shrinkage' include headaches, fatigue, confusion, dizziness and reduced concentration and cognition.
- It takes around 90 minutes of sweating either through physical activity or warm climate or a deficit in fluid intake of around 1 L a day to begin to affect brain function.
- Caffeine and alcohol are both diuretics and are common causes of brain shrinkage.
- Safe caffeine consumption is around 200 mg a day for adults, 90 mg a day for teenagers, and very little for children. This is equivalent to 2-3 cups of coffee or 3-4 cups of tea a day for adults and half this amount for teenagers.
- Caffeine is often hidden in food and drink products. Make sure you read labels well.
- Alcohol not only acts as a diuretic but also causes toxic effects on brain tissue if consumed in large amounts either on a regular basis or as a result of binge drinking.
- The safe alcohol limits currently accepted are 2 standard drinks a day 5 days a week with 2 alcohol-free days a week for adults. It can be very easy to drink more than this so ensure you understand the amount of alcohol in a standard drink by reading the label.

YOUR *Weekly* CHALLENGE . . . .

This week your aim is two-fold - reduce your caffeine intake to no more than 2-3 cups of coffee or 3-4 cups of tea per day and reduce your alcohol intake to no more than 2 standard drinks a day, with 2 alcohol-free days this week. Try to have a glass of water for every cup of coffee/tea or alcoholic drink you have. If you are finding it hard to reduce your alcohol intake consider drinking mineral water in a wine/champagne glass to make it feel 'special'.

simple health habit #4

sleep well

How much sleep do you get? Sleep is so vital for health and yet many of us try to get by with so little. Studies show that up to 1 in 3 Australians consistently do not get enough good-quality sleep[1]. This means that there are up to 7 million people walking around sleep deprived every day. It seems we are a nation of insomniacs!

Why Do You Need Sleep?

Sleep is essential for life. The longest scientifically recorded period without sleep was just over 11 days. The record holder reported hallucinations, paranoia, blurred vision, slurred speech and memory and concentration lapses[1]. Much less severe but similar symptoms occur when we have repeatedly disturbed sleep or not enough sleep. I have met many an insomniac who describes themselves as a 'walking zombie'. So why do we need sleep?

Sleep allows for several vital functions including:

- Repair of our tissues[2]
- Growth in children by stimulating release of a growth hormone[3]
- Control of body-fat levels and appetite by stimulating release of the hormone leptin (so a person that does not sleep well can have problems controlling their body weight and appetite)[3]
- Slowing the ageing process[2]
- Boosting the immune system[3]
- Reducing stress hormone levels, which reduces depression, irritability, and anxiety[2]
- Improving concentration, alertness and brain function (studies have shown that 17 hours of sustained wakefulness leads to a decrease in performance equivalent to a blood alcohol level of 0.05 per cent[1])

Although we know that sleep is important, scientists are still not sure why we dream. Some scientists believe we dream to consolidate our long-term memory – that is, we dream about things worth remembering. Others have proposed we dream about things worth forgetting in order to eliminate overlapping memories that would otherwise fill up our brains during our waking hours.

How Much Sleep Do You Need?

Studies have shown that in order to ensure good health and longevity the amount of sleep required is about 7-9 hours per night for adults[2]. Interestingly, prior to the electric light bulb adults slept an average of 9-10 hours per night in line with sunrise and sunset[1]. Some studies suggest women need up to an hour extra of sleep a night compared to men, and without this extra hour women are much more susceptible to depression than men[1].

How Do You Get Good Quality Sleep?

We sleep because of a hormone called melatonin. This hormone is released from a part of our brain called the pineal gland when we are exposed to darkness. Hence we can disrupt melatonin production by being exposed to bright lights. Melatonin starts to rise about 2 hours before bedtime and regulates our sleep cycles.

Health FACT . . . .

You know you are not getting enough sleep at night if you consistently fall asleep within 5 mins. The ideal is between 10 to 15 minutes to fall asleep.

Sleep is actually not one long period of unconsciousness but, rather, consists of different states of sleep that move through a cycle during the night. These sleep cycles are regular alternations between deeper sleep and lighter REM (rapid eye movement) sleep. Each cycle takes about 90 minutes to complete, and the cycle repeats 4-5 times across a normal sleep period. This cyclic nature of sleep is present at all ages. How you feel when you wake, and if you remember your dreams will depend on where you wake within the cycle. If you wake shortly after REM sleep you will recall your dreams vividly, even if you recall them only transiently and then forget what you dreamed about. You are also likely to feel disoriented and drowsy. There are personal devices and phone apps now available that allow you to monitor your quality of sleep. Although these have not been fully tested for accuracy, many of my patients have found them helpful in gauging the quality of their sleep.

healthy habits: 52 ways to better health

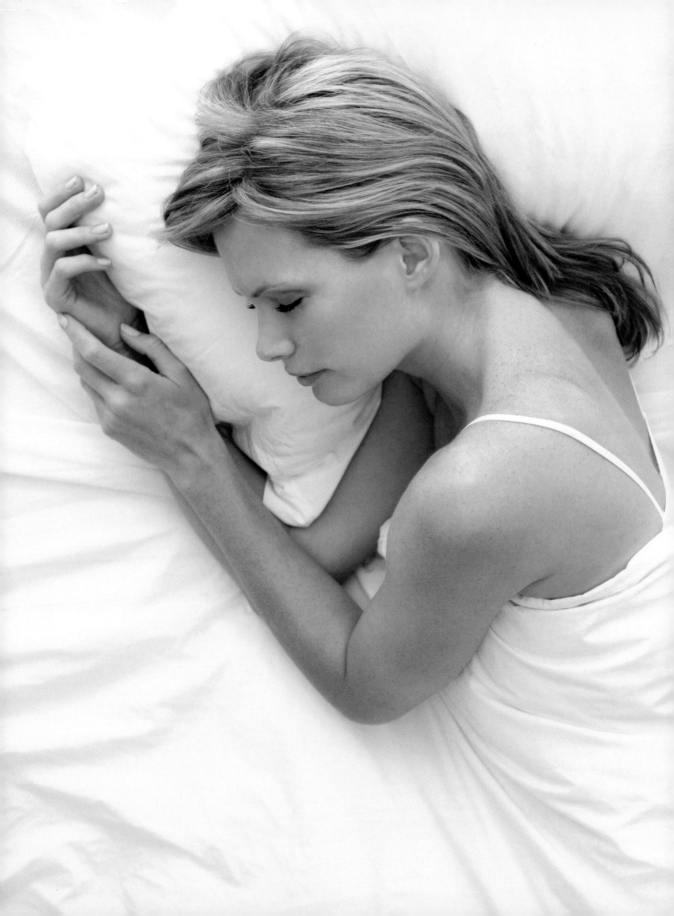

How Can You Ensure You Get a Good Night's Sleep?

Make sure your room is cool, dark, and quiet - around 18-22 degrees is considered the ideal, temperature as is a room that is pitch black, which encourages maximal melatonin production. A room that is quiet is best for undisturbed sleep. If your partner snores consider using ear plugs to reduce noise exposure.

- Remove electronic devices from the bedroom - the light emitted from these devices disrupts the production of melatonin.
- Do not turn on the bathroom light in the middle of the night. Consider buying a dim night light to help you see where you are going.
- Do not take work to bed with you - this increases stress-hormone production, which in turn reduces melatonin production.
- Reduce the time you spend co-sleeping with children and pets.
- Wind down in the evening by dimming the lights, keeping a peaceful environment and stopping work 1-2 hours before bed.
- Avoid caffeine and drinking excessive liquids 3-4 hours before bed.
- Avoid excessive alcohol before bed - although a sedative, alcohol disrupts quality of sleep by causing you to wake when blood-alcohol levels start to fall.
- Practise relaxation techniques regularly e.g. meditation, mindfulness, deep breathing.

Further to this, going to bed earlier is better than going to bed later, even if we get the same amount of sleep. This is because sleep quality has been scientifically shown to be best in the early hours of the evening[4].

How Do You Know If You Are Sleeping Well?

To diagnose a sleeping disorder the best way is to conduct a sleep study. This can now be done in the privacy of your own home where you are monitored for disturbed sleep during the night. The results can be very revealing.

I recall a male patient of mine who was always falling asleep in the afternoons when he got home from work. When he was at work he had no problem because he was kept busy, but as soon as he got home and sat himself in front of the television he was straight off to sleep within several minutes. This concerned him and his wife - he wanted to help out a little more with the kids, but found he just did not have the energy. He reported a full night's sleep most nights, which puzzled him because he was still exhausted the next day when he woke up. When we undertook a sleep study it revealed that he was actually waking up around 300 times per night! He was not even aware of this. At times he would even stop breathing during his sleep, which was concerning. This condition is called sleep apnoea and is quite common.

Could It Be Sleep Apnoea?

If you snore consider whether you may have sleep apnoea. Around 10 per cent of snorers suffer from this condition[5], which is a disorder that causes sufferers to wake – often up to hundreds of times per night – and even periodically stop breathing. Sleep apnoea significantly increases the risk of heart disease, stroke, enlarged heart, depression, high blood pressure, and even sudden death[5]. If you snore it is worth making an appointment with your GP to rule out sleep apnoea.

Do You Still Feel Tired?

If you are waking up from a night's sleep still tired it may be time for a medical check-up. Common conditions that lead to fatigue:

- Sleep apnoea
- Sleep disorders
- Anxiety and/or depression
- High stress-hormone levels
- Anaemia or other blood disorders
- Low and/or imbalanced sex hormones
- Thyroid conditions
- Autoimmune conditions
- Malignancies

Can You Catch Up on 'Sleep Debt'?

Getting too little sleep creates a 'sleep debt', which is like being overdrawn at a bank. Eventually, your body will demand that the debt be repaid. We don't seem to adapt to getting little sleep; while we may get used to a sleep-depriving schedule, our judgment, reaction time and other functions are still impaired. You can catch up to some degree on lost sleep as long as the sleep debt is not too high. Consider recovering your sleep debt every few days by getting a good night's sleep.

What Can You Take to Improve Sleep?

Sometimes individuals need to take medication to help them get a good night's sleep. Sleeping medication can be prescribed or bought over the counter.

The most commonly prescribed sleeping medication is a group known as benzodiazepines which include temazepam[1]. The issue with these types of sleeping tablets is they do not allow a deep sleep but rather a transient, superficial sleep. This means that you are still likely to wake up feeling tired. The long-term risk of taking benzodiazepines is that you may become physically dependent on the drugs and find it difficult to sleep without them. To limit the chance of dependence take only on alternating nights, or three times a week, and at the lowest effective dose possible for a limited time e.g. a month[1].

The other common medication available on prescription in Australia, and over the counter in other countries, is the sleep hormone melatonin. Much like your body's natural melatonin, the prescribed version acts to reset your body clock. Melatonin has been shown to be effective in treating insomnia in many people, particularly among people aged over 55 years. It is worth trying 2-5 mg daily as a slow-release tablet or liquid if you are having difficulties with insomnia and/or you are a shift worker or travel overseas and need to reset your body clock[1].

If you prefer natural remedies, there is evidence showing that valerian can mildly improve sleep[1]. Purchase a good-quality product so that you know the ingredients are as pure as possible.

Take Home Points

Sleep is essential for health and life.

- Adults need on average 7-9 hours sleep per night.
- The best quality sleep is before midnight.
- Practise good techniques to ensure a restful night's sleep – do not take work to bed with you, keep the room cool, dark and quiet, and reduce exposure to artificial lighting and screens at least one hour before bed.
- Recognise if you have sleep apnoea and consider having a full medical check-up if you are consistently feeling tired when you wake in the mornings.
- Catch up on 'sleep debt' regularly.
- Limit the use of sleeping medication to avoid tolerance and dependence. Try natural substances such as melatonin and valerian first.

YOUR *Weekly* CHALLENGE . . . .

This week your aim is to get enough good-quality sleep on most nights. Aim to go to bed by 10 p.m. at the latest.

rest & recover

There is a big difference between 'sleep' and 'rest and recovery'. Rest involves allowing our bodies and minds to be free from anxiety, worry and stress. Recovery is similar but goes even further in that it involves recognising our body's cues for when we need to stop and allow our tissues to re-energise and repair.

Many of us are under the impression that we have unlimited energy reserves with no need to rest and recover at all. Alternatively, even if we recognise the need to rest or recover, we have no margin in our schedule to allow this to happen. Too often I see individuals running into trouble with burn-out as a result of not resting and recovering.

What Is Burn-Out?

Burn-out is a state where our bodies and minds are incapable of functioning well. Unfortunately, few burn-out sufferers see it coming until it's too late. If you, however, identify signs of burn-out early enough, you can reverse the downward spiral. According to psychologist and author Sherrie Bourg Carter, the typical features of burn-out include[1]:

- Physical and emotional exhaustion
- Feelings of cynicism and detachment
- A sense of ineffectiveness and lack of accomplishment

Together these symptoms lead to an inability to function successfully on a personal and professional level. The problem with allowing ourselves to get to this state is that it can take a long time to recover.

How You Can Avoid Burn-Out

There are some key steps to avoiding burn-out. Firstly, throughout the day, recognise when your energy levels are waning e.g. restlessness, yawning, hunger and difficulty concentrating. Studies have shown that our minds and bodies need a break from work every 90 to 120 minutes throughout the day[2]. Try taking some deep breaths, stretching, and/or take a brisk walk around the block for 10 minutes. Even just shutting your eyes and meditating for a brief period is enough to restore your concentration. Other strategies to avoid burn-out include:

- Practising mindfulness throughout the day (explained on page 38)
- Taking a power nap (explained on page 38)
- Trying the relaxation technique described on page 37
- Eating regularly to avoid low blood-sugar dips
- Avoiding excessive amounts of caffeine, which deplete energy reserves quickly
- Designating an end point to your day e.g. a 'clock-off' time beyond which you do not do any more work
- Taking regular holidays. Studies have shown that regular short breaks such as a weekend away can be just as rejuvenating as a longer holiday. Interestingly, holidays that are longer than 9 days add no more benefits in terms of rejuvenation than those that are up to 9 days long. So the key, really, is to take breaks often. I recommend taking a break every 8-12 weeks even if it is for a weekend.
- Trying not to bring work home with you
- Creating a routine in the evening for winding down. This might involve reading the paper, having a bath or reading a book
- Prioritising enjoyable activities that are not work-related in your week. This might be a sport, going shopping or even just watching a movie
- Seeking professional guidance if experiencing signs of burn-out

So burn-out is essentially avoidable if you recognise your early warning signs and take proactive measures to halt it progressing. Perhaps trying the relaxation technique below at least once throughout your day will help.

Health TIP . . . .

Our minds and bodies function best when we have a short break from work every 90 to 120 minutes.

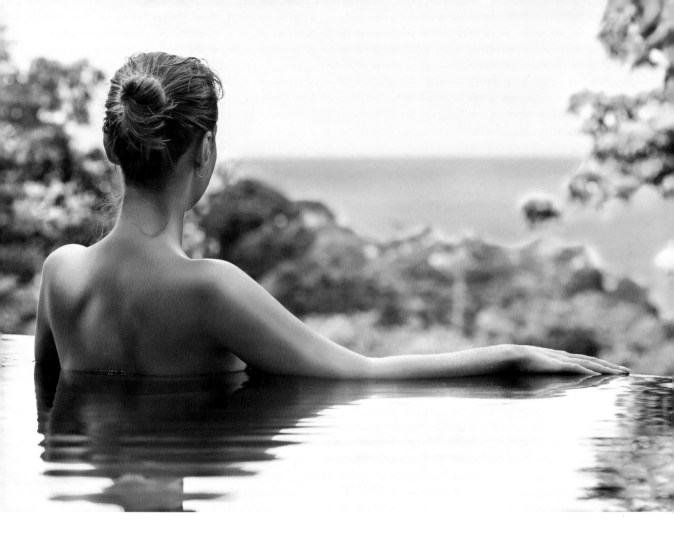

Quick Relaxation Break

Try this 5-minute relaxation technique which can be practised any time or place for a quick refresh.

Step 1 Sit or lie in a comfortable position.

Step 2 Put your hands on your abdomen and, as you breathe in, let your abdomen expand like a balloon filling with air.

Step 3 As you exhale, slowly let the air out. You should feel your abdomen rising and falling as you breathe.

Step 4 Try to raise your shoulders up to your ears for 5 seconds, and then let your shoulders drop. One at a time, rotate each shoulder backward 5–10 times, and then rotate them together 5–10 times.

Step 5 In a relaxed position, close your eyes and breathe naturally. Count to 4 as you inhale, then pause for 1 count, then exhale for 4 counts.

Step 6 Continue this for at least 5 minutes.

Another great long-term strategy to avoid burn-out is to learn and practise the art of mindfulness.

How You Can Be Mindful

Mindfulness is a form of self-awareness training adapted from mindfulness meditation. Mindfulness is about being aware of what is happening in the present on a moment-by-moment basis, while not making judgements about whether we like or do not like what we find. We all have the capacity to be mindful. It simply involves cultivating our ability to pay attention in the present moment and allows us to disengage from mental 'clutter' and to have a clear mind. It makes it possible for us to respond rather than react to situations, thus improving our decision-making and potential for physical and mental relaxation.[3]

In 1993 psychologist Marsha Linehan articulated some components of being mindful[4]. Firstly she described three 'what' skills:

- Observing (simply attending to events and emotions)
- Describing (applying matter-of-fact labels to emotions and situations)
- Participating (entering into current activities with full concentration)
  Secondly she described three 'how' skills:
- Taking a 'non-judgemental' stance
- Focussing on one thing in the moment
- Being effective (doing what is needed rather than worrying about what is right or second-guessing the situation)

Like anything worth developing, mindfulness takes practice to master in our everyday lives. Consider undertaking a 5-minute online mindfulness tutorial to incorporate this way of thinking into your busy daily schedule.

Another strategy to avoid burn-out is to power nap throughout the day whenever you get the opportunity.

Harness the Power of a 'Power Nap'

Perhaps countries like Spain have the right idea by incorporating siestas into their daily routines. After all, performance has been shown to increase by 34 per cent following a power nap[4]! Researchers have found that people are designed to have 2 sleeps per day – the main one at night and a nap in the afternoon[4]. Cortisol, the hormone responsible for alertness as well as stress, naturally starts to decline at about 2–3 p.m. leading to the 'afternoon slump'. Having a short power nap of 20 minutes allows our energy and alertness levels to pick up again. Even very successful individuals like Winston Churchill, Albert Einstein, and Thomas Edison were known to power nap regularly.

So what are some tips for power napping?

- Lie undisturbed in a comfortable chair or couch for 20–30 minutes. Even if you don't actually fall asleep the 'rest' will still have a positive effect.
- Try not to lie down in bed during the day. Save this for night-time rest so that you don't oversleep during the day.
- Make the room as dark as possible.
- Make the room temperature comfortable.
- Switch off technology.
- Try not to sleep too close to bedtime as this might interfere with night-time sleep.
- Don't feel guilty for resting.

So, to sum up, power napping can be a powerful tool to improve productivity and performance. Realistically you may only be able to achieve a power nap 1–2 times per week, but this will still be of benefit.

Burn-out is a huge problem in our society. It can affect anyone at any given time in their lives. The key to overcoming burn-out is to recognise when you are heading towards it and to pull back and truly rest and recover. It is better to be proactive in avoiding burn-out than find yourself in the doctor's surgery completely debilitated.

Take Home Points

Rest and recovery is important to avoid burn-out.

- Key features of burn-out include physical and emotional exhaustion, feelings of cynicism and detachment, and having a sense of ineffectiveness and lack of accomplishment at work and/or in your personal life.
- To avoid burn-out consider taking regular breaks throughout your day as well as regular holidays.
- Practising relaxation techniques, mindfulness and power napping regularly may also help with preventing burn-out.
- Always seek professional advice if you feel that you are headed for burn-out as this can quickly spiral downwards and become debilitating.

YOUR *Weekly* CHALLENGE . . . .

This week your aim is to rest and recover every 90–120 minutes when you are working. This could involve a 5-minute break consisting of deep breathing, meditation, walking or stretching.

restore your biorhythms

Our bodies are finely in tune with certain environmental and internal cues. These cues set our biorhythms. When our biorhythms are functioning as they should, we are able to sleep well, our tissues are able to heal, our appetite is controlled, our body-fat stores are kept at bay, and our hormones are released in the correct amounts and at the most effective times of the day. When our biorhythms are not well regulated, however, our bodies do not function as efficiently and effectively as they could. The result is a range of symptoms that can be quite debilitating. Luckily there are some simple ways we can restore our biorhythms.

Health FACT . . . .

Restoring your natural biorhythms is key to having a good night's sleep, feeling energetic and controlling your appetite.

So What Exactly Is a Biorhythm?

In our body there are several 'body clocks' that are functioning often simultaneously throughout the day. These clocks are known as biorhythms or circadian rhythms and refer to the cycles of physiological and biological processes that fluctuate on a roughly 24-hour timetable. You have probably noticed these cycles yourself, feeling more energetic and alert during peak periods of the day and more lethargic and run down at other times of the day. Another example is that mental alertness tends to peak twice in a day, at 9 a.m. and 9 p.m., while physical strength tends to crest at 11 a.m. and 7 p.m.

While we all have circadian rhythms there are differences in the length of the cycles, which helps to explain why some of us are 'night owls' and others are 'morning people'.

There also appears to be a genetic component to our rhythms, which explains why lifestyle habits such as staying up late appear to run in some families and not in others. The image below shows many of the biorhythms at work in our bodies every day.

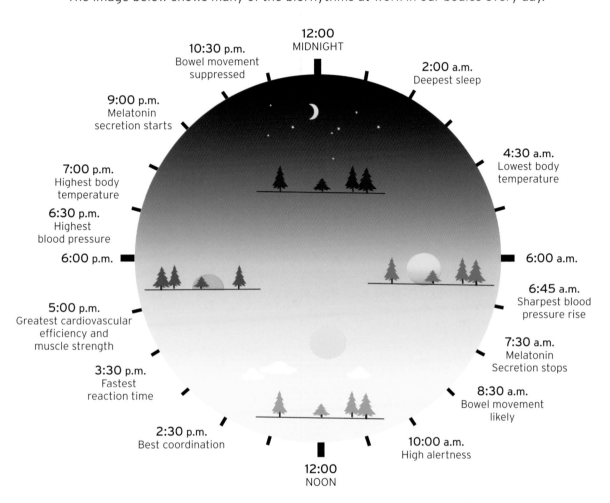

From the image we can see that melatonin secretion, body temperature, vascular changes and bowel changes, amongst other things, fluctuate throughout the day as part of our biorhythms. To highlight this further let us focus on melatonin, our sleep hormone, which is released somewhere between 9 p.m. and 7:30 a.m. This sets in place our natural sleep cycle. For those of us who work late hours or night shifts we are in direct contention with this natural cycle and this may lead to issues with sleep or other aspects of our health.

One of the worst work situations I have found myself in was when I was undertaking alternating night and day shifts at a hospital. No sooner would my body clock get used to a night-time routine than I would have to switch to a day shift and vice versa. I would constantly feel tired, have no appetite yet was gaining weight and had great difficulty sleeping when I was meant to. After a while I found that my mood started deteriorating and looking back on the situation I was probably bordering on depression. The best thing I felt I could do in that situation was to not alternate day and night shifts but rather request extended periods of day shifts followed by night shifts and so on. This way I was granted at least 3-4 weeks at a time to get used to a new routine and my biorhythms would have time to adjust.

What Influences Your Biorhythms?

Our biorhythms are very much in tune with environmental cues as well as internal body cues, but the greatest influence on our biorhythms is exposure to sunlight. Regular exposure to sunlight during waking hours helps to set our biorhythms. Other influences on our biorhythms include when we eat, when we sleep, when we are most active and whether we are exposed to artificial lighting. Our modern-day lifestyles have altered our usual practices to the point where we are no longer in tune with internal body cues, which have become confused with our body's response to artificial external cues.

How Do You Know If Your Biorhythms Are Out of Balance?

When our biorhythms are not functioning well we can experience a range of symptoms including:

- Sleep disruption
- Difficulty falling asleep
- Increased appetite
- Difficulty losing weight
- Not healing quickly following an injury, illness or period of intense exercise
- Reduced concentration

A growing body of research has suggested that disrupted biorhythms may increase the chance of cardiovascular complications such as heart attacks, as well as obesity and neurological problems like depression and bipolar disorder.

How Can You Restore Your Biorhythms?

The best way to strengthen our biorhythms is to strengthen our 'zeitgebers'. It was German Scientist Jurgen Aschoff who first coined the term zeitgeber, which translated means 'time-keeper' or 'synchroniser'. What Aschoff found was that our body actually synchronises to certain cues afforded by routine. Although we may often resist routine in favour of being flexible with our schedules, our body actually needs routine to set its biorhythms. Routine timing for some key events throughout the day helps to establish

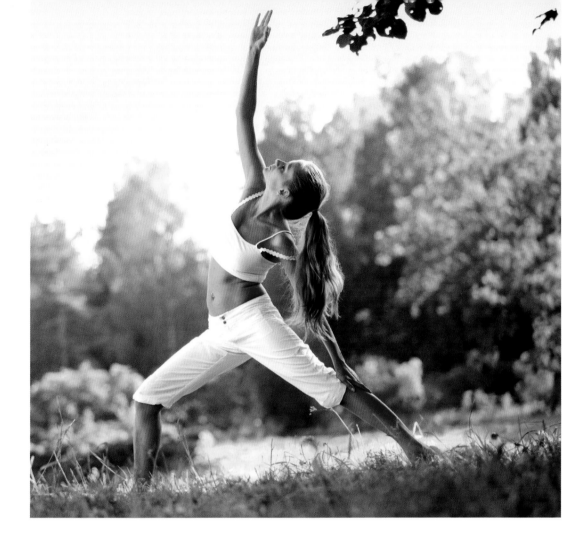

a predictable pattern of hormone release and helps to set our body clocks. These key synchronisers or zeitgebers include:

- Attempting to go to bed at the same time each night
- Waking up at the same time each morning
- Eating at roughly the same times each day
- Avoiding eating at unusual times, including very late at night
- Exercising at the same times each day
- Getting some natural sunlight exposure each day

These key events reinforce the body's natural sleep-awake cycle and the biorhythms that are intertwined with our sleep-awake cycle. Now if this seems too strict, the steps to try at a minimum are to wake at the same time each morning and to get some natural sunlight exposure each day. These two steps alone will go a long way in strengthening your biorhythms.

This also works if you are travelling and need to reset your body clock to a new time zone. Simply re-establish a daily schedule based on these activities in your new time zone. After just a few days of being consistent with your new routine your body clock, and therefore biorhythms, will reset and in turn you will avoid extended jet lag. The same goes for restoring your biorhythms even if you are not travelling. Simply strengthen your zeitgebers and be consistent with the above activities and within a few days your body clock will be set. The result is waking feeling refreshed, having an appetite that is under control, bowel motions that come at regular times, and feeling less fatigued throughout the day.

Take Home Points

Our biorhythms are natural cycles that are at work in us continuously.

- Many of our hormones are released in response to our biorhythms.
- When our biorhythms are disrupted we may feel fatigued, have difficulty getting a good night's sleep, have a change in our appetite and bowel motions, find it difficult to lose weight, have difficulty concentrating, and even find that we feel despondent or depressed.
- Our biorhythms can be disrupted by not getting enough sunlight throughout the day, by having an inconsistent routine, by not getting enough sleep and by being exposed to artificial lighting close to bedtime.
- To strengthen our biorhythms we need to establish a consistent daily routine. This involves going to bed at the same time each night, waking at the same time each morning, eating at the same times throughout the day and exercising at the same times each day.
- It usually takes around 3 days to reset your body clock (after travelling, for instance), but it can take up to 7 days.
- The result of restoring or establishing your biorhythms is waking feeling refreshed, having an appetite that is under control, bowel motions that come at regular times, and feeling less fatigued throughout the day.

YOUR *Weekly* CHALLENGE . . . .

This week your challenge is to restore your biorhythms by trying to establish a consistent routine whereby every day this week you go to bed at the same time, wake at the same time, eat at around the same times, and exercise at the same times throughout the day.

eat by the 80/20 rule

With medical and scientific knowledge constantly being updated there is often confusion regarding which foods are good for us and which to avoid. It even sometimes seems like experts contradict themselves. But one principle will always stand: unprocessed, wholesome foods such as fresh fruits, vegetables and wholegrains will always be healthier for us than processed foods such as chips, pastries, processed meats and sugary snacks. Balance is the key, as with anything in life, and so I like to prescribe eating by the 80/20 rule.

Health FACT . . . .

Unprocessed, wholesome foods contain the vital nutrients, minerals, vitamins, antioxidants and fibre our body needs to function well.

By this I mean that 80 per cent of your daily diet ideally should be made up of unprocessed, wholesome foods. These foods come in their own original packaging made by nature – peels, skins, shells or outer leaves. They either grow in the ground, grow on trees, or come from animals. They are not processed, do not contain artificial flavours, colours, preservatives or sweeteners. These are the foods that are ideal for human consumption and lead to good health. They provide the nutrients, antioxidants, vitamins and minerals needed to protect us from chronic diseases. They also give us energy rather than steal energy from us. In essence this should be our fuel source most of the time.

The other 20 per cent of our diet can be made up of the other foods we enjoy in moderation including the high sugar, salty and fatty foods, as well as alcohol. In small amounts these types of foods are fine but in large amounts they can make you disease-prone, cause diabetes, heart disease and strokes, and can make you overweight. In large quantities these types of foods will also make you fatigued and prone to high blood pressure and high cholesterol. Sadly, many people consume food in the opposite way to the ratio and eat mostly processed foods and very little fresh, wholesome produce.

I would often share this principle at The Biggest Loser Retreat, when I worked there as the health consultant, with mixed responses. Often there was a sense of relief that the secret to eating healthily could be simplified to one basic principle, there was disbelief that eating healthily could really be so simple. It doesn't need to be overcomplicated and difficult – just following the 80/20 rule when it comes to making food choices is a major positive step in the right direction. If we overcomplicate or over restrict our diet we risk becoming overwhelmed and may give up trying.

Let us now look at the specific components that would make up the healthy 80 per cent of our diet. These components are the 'macronutrients' our body needs, and contain vitamins, minerals, antioxidants and fibre.

Essential Components of Healthy Eating

Fruits and vegetables It is an established fact that the more fruits and vegetables we eat the lower our chance of heart disease, cancer and many other health problems. Try as best you can to buy fresh, seasonal produce rather than frozen or canned. Saying that, if you have to make a choice between eating frozen/canned vegetables/fruit or no vegetables/fruit due to budget constraints or remote location then of course you would choose the former. Try and eat vegetables lightly steamed or raw (not fried), because food in its natural state has all its enzymes. Enzymes are the chemical spark plugs in our bodies that start or speed up the chemical processes that help our bodies with things like digestion. No fruit or vegetable is better than another. Enjoy all kinds and eat a variety.

Starches Starches contain carbohydrates and include grains and starchy vegetables such as potato, corn, carrots, peas and sweet potato, as well as legumes and beans. Our bodies need carbohydrates to create energy and a sense of well-being, but in excess they can raise our insulin levels, which can eventually lead to Type 2 Diabetes. Choose unprocessed varieties such as wholegrain breads, whole-wheat pasta, quinoa, millet, amaranth, buckwheat and brown Basmati or Dongara rice. Avoid eating too many 'white' starches, including white bread, white rice, pastries, biscuits and crackers made from white flour. When baking opt for wholemeal flour, almond meal, spelt or coconut flour.

Dairy Do choose unsweetened dairy products such as plain Greek yoghurt rather than flavoured. Limit cheese to occasional serves of hard and soft cheeses and opt instead for ricotta, cottage or feta cheese. As for milk, I do not recommend drinking

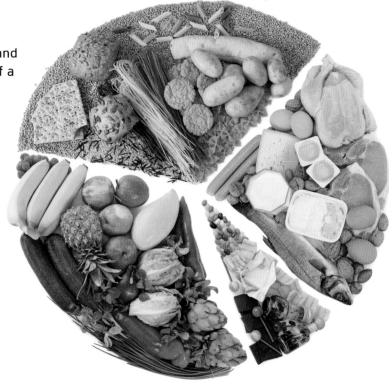

Components and Proportions of a Healthy Diet

unpasteurised milk as this has been linked to potentially life-threatening conditions especially for the young, elderly, pregnant and sick. Some individuals find they can better digest A2 milk and others do better on lactose-free milk. Both of these are fine to drink. If you are intolerant to all dairy choose unsweetened rice, oat, almond or soy milk. There is some concern that soy milk may lead to problems with thyroid function after long-term use. Due to this concern limit soy milk to occasional use and opt for one of the other dairy-free alternatives. If you are dairy intolerant, other sources of high-calcium foods include tinned sardines, tinned salmon, broccoli and green leafy vegetables such as spinach and bok choy.

Protein Try cutting down on processed meats like salami and packaged meat slices, which can contain high-levels of cancer-causing agents known as nitrosamines. Opt instead for hormone-free, free-range chicken, turkey, beef, lamb, or fresh fish. Grill, bake, steam, boil or lightly stir-fry your meat rather than smoke, chargrill or barbeque as these processes have been linked with increased risk of bowel cancer. Avoid shark (flake) and swordfish as they have some of the highest levels of mercury and pesticides of any fish. Men, limit your intake of red meat as men who consume high amounts of red meat double or triple their chances of developing prostate cancer.

Eggs Eggs are a good source of protein and contain plenty of vitamins and minerals, as well as beneficial substances like choline, needed for cell-membrane synthesis, and lutein, needed for protection of our eyes. Eggs were once thought to greatly elevate cholesterol levels but this does not seem to be the case. I recommend eating around 4–6 eggs per week. Do choose free-range or organic eggs, which often have a higher omega-3 content than caged chicken eggs. Boil or poach your eggs rather than fry them.

Fats Have some good fats in your diet as your body needs some fat to survive. The right type of fats in the right amounts is important for your heart, brain, skin, hair and hormone production. Include a small amount of healthy fats found in avocados, cold-pressed extra-virgin olive oil, nuts and seeds, as well as in oily fish like salmon, tuna, herring, mackerel and sardines. Keep in mind that tuna, especially the larger yellow-fin tuna, contains higher levels of mercury than other oily fish, so limit this particular variety.

Also keep in mind that olive oil is not the best oil to cook with as it has a low smoke point; meaning that when used for cooking at high heat it quickly starts to smoke and produce some toxic chemicals that have been linked to cancer formation. Save olive oil for adding to your salads or vegetables as a dressing and cook instead with oils that have a high smoke point. These oils include grape seed oil, rice bran oil, macadamia nut oil and avocado oil.

Take Home Points

Eating healthily does not need to be complicated.

- Follow the 80/20 rule when it comes to making food choices.
- 80 per cent of the foods you eat in any given day should be unprocessed, wholesome foods such as fresh fruits and vegetables, plain unsweetened dairy or dairy alternatives, wholegrain starches, lean meats, eggs and good fats.
- The other 20 per cent of the foods you eat can be foods you enjoy in moderation that may be processed and thus made from white flour and/or contain high amounts of sugar, salt and fat.

YOUR *Weekly* CHALLENGE . . . .

This week your challenge is to eat by the 80/20 rule. Choose mainly unprocessed, wholesome foods including fresh fruits and vegetables, plain unsweetened dairy or dairy alternatives, eggs, lean meats, wholegrains, beans, legumes, and nuts and seeds.

clean out your pantry

Cleaning out your pantry is key to improving your health. Simply by making sure we have healthy food staples at hand and minimal temptation in the house means we can stay on track with our health goals. Sometimes we feel that we need to keep snack foods in the pantry for the kids or other family members. This often creates unnecessary tension between what we want to eat and what is available. If there are less healthy food choices kept in the home then more often than not in a moment of fatigue, upset or boredom we will make the wrong choice. My suggestion would be to take some time to clean out the pantry. Try not to worry about wasting food. Donate your unwanted food items to a charity food drive. Clearing out the pantry will be of benefit to the whole family as healthier snack alternatives are sought and eaten in place of highly processed foods. Employing the help of family members and explaining to them the importance of eating healthily may help resolve any resistance to clearing out the pantry.

Health FACT

Keeping foods that cause temptation out of the house means you are less likely to make poor food choices.

On page 50 is a list of pantry staples to which all other food items can be made. Top up your pantry weekly with these staples. Buying in bulk sometimes means saving money, too, so look for weekly shopping bargains and stock up on non-perishable items that may be on sale.

Pantry Staples

- Wholegrain, spelt or rye bread (not whole*meal*, which is still high-glycaemic index. Avoid low-glycaemic index white breads, which are still highly processed).
- Flat breads such as Mountain Bread. Not only are they great for wraps, but they can also be used to make lasagne and quiches in place of filo pastry.
- Wholegrains (brown rice, Basmati, Dongara, wild, pearl barley, burghal)
- Wholemeal pasta (or buckwheat pasta if gluten intolerant/allergic)
- Canned corn (no added sugar or salt)
- Canned beans and lentils (unsalted)
- Dried lentils
- Plain rice cakes or corn thins
- Plain rice crackers
- Wholegrain crispbreads such as Ryvita®
- Fruit-free wholegrain muesli bars such as Carman's Fruit Free
- Plain rolled oats and/or wholegrain cereals such as the Goodness Superfoods range
- Wholemeal plain and self-raising flour
- Bicarbonate soda
- Herbs and spices (any variety, but do choose cinnamon without added sugar)
- Pink Himalayan sea salt (the least processed and has the most minerals, including iodine, which many women are deficient in, which can lead to thyroid issues)
- Vanilla essence (without added sugar)
- Unsalted raw nuts (all except peanuts have health benefits)
- Chicken or vegetable stock (preservative and MSG free) such as Massel brand
- Cooking oil such as rice bran oil, macadamia oil, avocado oil, coconut oil or grapeseed oil (these have a high smoke point)
- Olive oil as a salad dressing
- Apple cider vinegar and/or balsamic vinegar as a dressing
- Plain, minimally sweetened biscuits (ideally trans fat free)
- Xylitol and/or stevia
- Raw cacao (can be used to add chocolate flavour to baking and making other snacks without adding the sugar and unhealthy fats)
- Good quality protein powder such as brown-rice protein, pea protein or whey isolate (if not dairy intolerant). This can be used to make protein shakes and protein balls for a snack

- Popping corn for movie nights or as a healthy snack
- Canned salmon and tuna (but be aware that tuna can have high levels of mercury. Limit tuna to once a week and choose mostly salmon, which has a lower mercury content. Smaller tuna have lower amounts of mercury if you can find them on your supermarket shelves. Look for Tungol tuna)
- Unsalted pretzels
- Black tea, herbal teas and coffee (aim for plain instant coffee rather than flavoured and sweetened varieties. Also, if choosing decaffeinated coffee keep in mind to buy either organic or water-filtered decaffeinated rather than standard decaffeinated, which is chemically produced)
- Red wine (ideally preservative-free. Red wine has the most health benefits while beer has the least)
- Psyllium husks to add to breakfast cereal or a protein shake for added fibre
- Keep in mind that items that are labelled gluten-free are not always that healthy for us. Often they are refined, white-rice products, which have a very high glycaemic index. A better choice is to look for wholegrain gluten-free products such as those containing millet, buckwheat, amaranth and brown rice.

Avoid keeping highly processed foods in the pantry such as potato chips, flavoured biscuits and lollies. It is worth also clearing out the fridge and freezer and replacing items that are not that healthy with alternatives. Below is a list of fridge and freezer staples.

Freezer Staples

- Frozen berries (good for baking with as well as in smoothies)
- Frozen white fish and salmon (unflavoured and unbattered)
- Frozen steam-fresh vegetables

Fridge Staples

- Fresh milk (choose A2 milk if you find that digestion is a problem. If you find dairy still causes issues trial lactose-free milk, unsweetened almond milk or rice milk. Avoid soy milk if you can as there is some suggestion that too much soy may cause issues with hormone and thyroid imbalances)
- Butter instead of margarine (choose unsalted butter and avoid margarine, which is highly processed)
- A wide range of fresh vegetables and fruits

- Unsweetened yoghurt such as Greek yoghurt
- Hummus (make sure it is preservative-free or make your own)
- Almond spread (instead of peanut butter spread)
- Ricotta, cottage or fetta cheese instead of block cheeses, soft cheeses or processed cheese)
- Eggs (free-range, organic and, if you can find them, omega-3 eggs are best)
- Ham and/or turkey for sandwiches (nitrate free is best)
- Fresh fish (avoid bass, swordfish and flake as these are high in mercury content)
- Fresh seafood such as shellfish, oysters and prawns (limit these to once per week due to high natural cholesterol content)
- Chicken breast, tenderloins and/or thighs (choose free-range, hormone-free or organic)
- Lean beef (hormone-free)
- Lamb (hormone-free)
- Mineral water, soda water or tonic water (to make spritzers or as a variation on plain water)
- Dark chocolate (ideally buy small snack sizes rather than large family blocks)

Avoid dressings, sauces, mayonnaise, soft drinks and cordials. Instead of jams try almond spread or avocado.

Superfoods – Are They Really That Super?

Superfoods claim to be saviours of health, and include, but are not limited to, goji berries, flaxseed, acai berries, chia seeds, spirulina and barley grass. It would seem that even when our diet is a little off kilter when it comes to making healthy choices, we can simply add a bit of spirulina here and some goji berries there and all is redeemed.

At most, these will only make a small difference to your health. The greatest difference will come from all the other strategies mentioned in this book. Consider at this stage just adding as many of these 'superfoods' to your diet as your budget allows.

Should You Eat Organic?

Organic produce is grown without the use of chemicals or pesticides. It is claimed that organic produce is cultivated the way nature intended. There is no doubt that organic produce tends to contain more vitamins and minerals than non-organic due to more traditional farming practices that focus on the quality of growing soils. Furthermore the lack of agricultural chemicals potentially means less risk to our bodies from known and unknown health effects. Organic fruit also tends to be picked when ripe rather than be artificially, chemically ripened, which is the case with many non-organic fruit.

The downside is that organic produce can be expensive and hard to come by. Do not avoid fruit and vegetables because you are concerned about produce being non-organic. Where possible and where your budget allows purchase organic produce. Perhaps consider buying the items that cannot be peeled such as spinach, lettuce, tomatoes, berries, mushrooms, squash, and zucchini, the idea being that items that can be peeled will at least allow for removal of pesticide-laden skins. Wash produce well in a fruit and vegetable wash specifically created to remove pesticides. Often this is a natural detergent that can be found in most health food stores.

Take Home Points

Clear out the pantry, fridge and freezer and replace highly processed food items with fresh, unprocessed foods such as lean meats, fresh produce, fresh unsweetened dairy products, eggs, nuts, legumes and beans and wholegrains.

- Keep highly processed snacks out of the house. The rest of your family will benefit from this also, so don't feel guilty about 'depriving' other family members of the foods they want. Regardless of how much exercise someone does, how thin someone is, or how young, no one's health benefits from regularly consuming these sorts of snack foods.

- Add superfoods into your diet once the rest of your diet is looking healthy. Do not spend extra money on superfoods if the rest of your diet is mostly unhealthy as you will be wasting money.

- Purchase organic produce as your budget allows. Save on the cost of produce by choosing organic items that cannot be peeled. Wash produce well with a vegetable/ fruit wash that removes most of the agricultural pesticides. This wash can be purchased from most health food stores.

YOUR *Weekly* CHALLENGE . . . .

This week your challenge is to clean out your pantry, fridge, and freezer. Make a list of healthy food staples and fill your house with these instead of highly processed, unhealthy foods. Always having healthy food options in the house will avoid unnecessary temptation.

pack a healthy lunchbox

There is really no point making an effort to have a healthy breakfast and dinner when you have fast-food for lunch, sugary foods as snacks, or nibble at cheese and crackers, salted nuts or baked goods that you find in the staffroom. Planning and preparing your lunch and snacks ahead of time is imperative to staying on track with your health goals. So what are some healthy lunchbox options?

Health TIP . . . .

Being organised and packing a healthy lunchbox is key to staying on track with health goals.

Healthy Lunches

Avoid skipping lunch even though you may be busy and tempted to just have a piece of fruit or biscuit when you feel peckish. Lunch is an important meal and helps to curb your appetite when you get those afternoon cravings. Eating lunch will also help keep your energy levels up for the rest of the day, and provides an opportunity to meet your daily fruit and vegetable intake.

There are some general principles to keep in mind when making a healthy lunch:

- Firstly try to keep lunch as fresh as possible. Avoid processed, pre-package, or frozen meals.
- Always include salad or vegetables at lunchtime.

- For a dressing choose lemon juice, olive oil or apple cider vinegar. Balsamic vinegar is okay occasionally but is higher in sugar than the other vinegars. Avoid creamy dressings such as Caesar dressings and ranch dressings.

- Always include some protein with your lunch, which will keep you feeling full. This may include, for example, a hard-boiled egg, lentils, beans, tofu, lean chicken, beef, lamb, turkey, tuna, salmon or sardines.

- Avoid processed meats like salami, prosciutto, chorizo, smoked salmon, Devon and ham. Instead roast some beef, a turkey or a chicken, and finely slice.

- Add a small amount of avocado to your salad. Keep in mind that avocado is rich in good fats but is very energy dense so you only need a small amount.

- If adding cheese choose lower-fat feta or cottage cheese rather than hard cheeses.

- A salad sandwich is another option using the above fillings. Choose wholegrain bread rather than wholemeal or white bread. To save on the bread calories consider having an open sandwich with just one slice of bread. Avoid adding mayonnaise, BBQ sauce or tomato sauce to your sandwich. Use avocado instead and keep butter to a minimum. Season with a small amount of salt and pepper.

- A wholegrain wrap or tortilla is another option, with the lowest calorie choice being Mountain bread. Mountain Bread can also be used to replace the pastry in lasagne, moussaka, pasties and quiches.

- Wholegrain crackers such as Ryvita are another option, as is corn and brown rice cakes.

- Of course you can always bring healthy leftovers from the night before to have as lunch.

- Drink only water or a cup of tea or coffee at lunchtime (preferably away from your meals to avoid digestion disruption). Avoid juice, alcohol, soft drinks, sweetened iced teas and flavoured milks, which add unnecessary sugar and calories.

Now that we have looked at some healthy lunch options, what are some healthy snack options?

Healthy Snacks

Having healthy snack options at hand helps you to avoid the temptation to buy something sugary. Having a mid-morning and mid-afternoon snack helps to keep blood sugar levels stable and keeps your metabolism working.

As with healthy lunches choosing a healthy snack is easy if you follow some general principles:

- Try and include protein with snacks
- Avoid processed snacks, which are often high in fat, sugar and/or salt
- Avoid chips, flavoured crackers or processed cheese

Healthy options include:
- Plain yoghurt with berries and oats sprinkled on top
- A small handful of raw nuts (unsalted and not roasted)
- Plain rice crackers with hummus
- A boiled egg
- Vegetable sticks with homemade dip
- Protein balls made with almond meal, tahini, cocoa powder and xylitol, and rolled in desiccated coconut

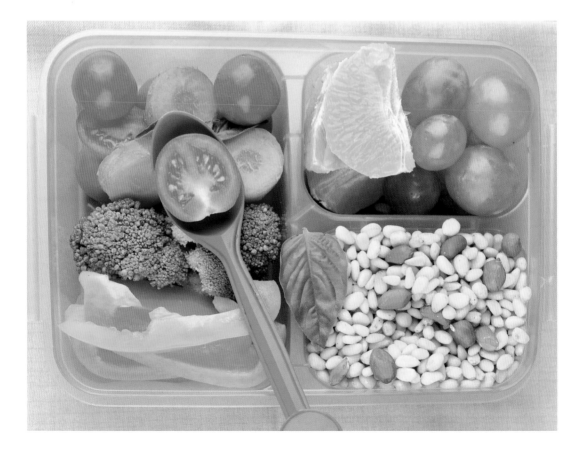

- Wholegrain crackers, corn thins or brown rice cakes with about 1-2 teaspoons of almond butter
- A protein shake made from ½ cup of almond milk, berries, 1 scoop whey isolate, rice protein or pea protein, 1 tsp ground flaxseed, and 1 tbsp psyllium husks
- If choosing muesli bars avoid those that are chocolate or yoghurt covered or have dried fruit and instead choose plain rolled-oat bars.

Another skill that you will need to master in order to keep up a healthy lifestyle is food-label reading. With more and more foods available already pre-prepared and packaged it can be difficult to know which are healthy options and which are laden with unwanted additives. So you need to look at the label carefully and be able to decipher all of those numbers.

How You Can Avoid Label Confusion

Label reading can be confusing but can be made easier by following a few basic principles.

On the back or sides of packets there will be three components to the food label:

1 One part of the food label is called the nutritional panel. This contains information about the Calories, macronutrients, salt (sodium), and occasionally vitamins. Avoid looking at the column that states 'per serving' as this can be deceptive. Some products will contain many serves per packet so you may eat the whole packet without realising that you have eaten two, three or more serves in one go and essentially all the Calories, fat, sugar etc. to go with it. Instead look at the column that states 'per 100 g' as this is the common comparator column between all products. Choose products that:
    - Contain less than 5 g per 100 g of total sugar
    - Contain less than 5 g per 100 g of saturated fat
    - Contain nil trans fats (more about trans fats later)
    - Contain less than 120 mg per 100 g of sodium

2 Often just underneath the nutritional panel is a list of potential allergens that may be found in the food product due to direct ingredients or due to the way the food was processed (for example, 'may contain nuts, dairy, gluten etc.'). If you are allergic or intolerant to these common food allergens then this is typically where you will find this information.

3 There will be a list, in order of amount added, of the ingredients of the product. Keep in mind that if the first three ingredients listed are sugar, fat, or salt avoid that product. It is likely to be a highly processed, energy-dense food item that will not be the healthiest choice.

balance your blood sugar

It is so important to balance our blood sugar levels. Blood sugar imbalances can cause a range of health symptoms and, as a clinician, I am seeing more and more of these problems arise. The other health concern with having unbalanced blood sugar levels long-term is something called 'insulin resistance', which can make it very difficult to lose weight, and eventually lead to type 2 diabetes. If you already have type 2 diabetes you can reduce the health damage caused by this disease by learning how to maintain stable blood sugar levels, as discussed in this chapter.

Health FACT

Around 280 Australians develop type 2 diabetes every day[1]. This illness is largely preventable by balancing blood sugar levels.

So What Are the Symptoms of Blood Sugar Problems?

Blood sugar imbalances can cause some significant symptoms in our bodies. These may be mild but in some cases can be debilitating. Warning signs that you may be experiencing blood sugar imbalances include:

- Feeling hungry only a few hours after you have eaten
- Feeling fatigued especially 1-2 hours after you have eaten
- Craving sugary foods
- Mood swings
- Waking in the middle of the night

- Not feeling satisfied with a meal
- Feeling faint, shaky, or dizzy
- Feeling hot and/or sweaty
- Gaining weight easily, especially tummy fat
- Having no energy to exercise
- Recurrent yeast infections
- Frequent urination or thirst (may be a sign of diabetes)

You may experience some or all of these symptoms and they can be present daily or just on occasion. The cure to reducing or eliminating these symptoms is to stabilise our blood sugar levels.

One particular patient comes to mind, a busy mother of three who was experiencing highs and lows of energy levels, mood swings, and an inability to lose weight especially from around her middle. When I examined her diet it was no wonder she was having these symptoms. She lived on the leftovers of her children's sugary breakfasts, snacks and dinners. She often skipped lunch and tide herself over with two to three cups of coffee. Her fluctuations in energy and moods were directly correlated to sugar spikes and dips. Once we made some adjustments to her diet by following some of the tips below she experienced a reduction in her symptoms and no longer felt like she 'was going crazy'.

Foods That Can Cause Blood Sugar Problems

Foods that cause blood sugar problems are those that have a high glycaemic index. Glycaemic index is a number given to foods that spike our blood sugar levels and, in turn, our insulin levels. When our insulin levels spike our body goes into overdrive to try and reduce our blood sugar levels back to normal. The problem is that this process can overshoot and what we are left with is a blood sugar level that has plummeted, with an energy level to match. Over time, constantly spiking our insulin levels can lead to storing body fat, insulin resistance, and eventually diabetes. Glycaemic index is designated to rank foods based on a number from 1 to 100. Those foods that rank less than 50 are those that will spike our blood sugar levels the least. Foods that are the highest in glycaemic index include:

- Most processed foods especially biscuits, cakes, pastries and most crackers
- Chips
- White rice
- Most gluten-free products made from potato or rice
- Most muesli bars
- Lollies and watery icy-poles

- White, wholemeal, Turkish and spelt breads
- Very sweet, low-fibre fruits such as watermelon, rockmelon and grapes
- White potato
- Fruit juice
- Soft drinks, cordials and iced tea
- Sugar, agave syrup, rice bran syrup and honey

Foods That Stabilise Blood Sugar Levels

Foods that have a glycaemic index of less than 50 help to stabilise blood sugar levels. They are absorbed slowly into our bloodstream and therefore do not spike our insulin levels. As a result we feel more satisfied with our meals, feel less hungry between meals, have fewer mood swings, and have higher sustained energy levels. Foods that help to stabilise blood sugar levels include:

- Bran, wholegrain cereals and bread
- Wholegrain gluten-free products (if gluten intolerant)
- Wholemeal pasta
- Basmati or Dongara rice (brown rice is still high glycaemic index but is less processed than white rice. If having brown rice mix with low glycaemic index vegetables)
- Wholegrain crackers
- Hummus or guacamole dip
- Fruits such as apples, pears, berries and oranges
- Vegetables other than white potato
- Yoghurt, smoothies and other dairy products (do choose unsweetened)
- Dark chocolate (do choose dark chocolate containing 70 per cent cocoa or more)

The key feature with all of these foods are that they are either high in fibre ('roughage') or contain protein such as dairy products. Look for foods that are higher in fibre and where possible eat the peel of fruits and vegetables. The peel adds roughage and therefore fibre, thus lowering the glycaemic index further.

Other Tips to Stabilise Your Blood Sugar Levels

Some practical strategies to stabilise your blood sugar levels include:

- Eating regular meals (every 3-4 hours).
- Eating protein with every meal, such as unsweetened yoghurt, nuts, hummus, legumes, tofu, chicken, meat or fish.

- Having a light snack before bed if it has been several hours between dinner and going to bed. This might include ½ a cup of unsweetened yoghurt and a piece of fruit or half a sandwich.
- Limit drinks to just water, tea (normal black tea and herbal) and coffee. Just a word on caffeine – this can cause spikes in your blood sugar due to release of sugar-releasing hormones. If you are having difficulties with blood sugar control consider limiting or eliminating caffeine for 3-5 days to see if you feel better.
- Limit daily sugar intake (discussed further below).

What Is So Bad About Sugar?

Most things in small amounts are not harmful. This is the same for sugar intake. The problem with excess sugar is that it is thought to:

Be addictive Sugar activates the pleasure centre in our brain much like other addictive substances.

Affect our appetite centre Sugar can cause people to feel hungry all the time.

Cause weight gain Through conversion to body fat due to the effects of insulin.

Predispose us to disease Heart disease, diabetes, gout, and can worsen polycystic ovaries.

Lead to bloating Bacteria in our intestines ferment undigested sugars.

So Where Does Sugar in Our Diet Come From?

Sugar is found in refined white sugar as well as naturally in fruits and many vegetables, honey, rice malt or bran syrup, coconut sugar, rapadura, molasses and agave syrup. It is often hidden in sauces, breakfast cereals and snack foods. The average Australian consumes around 60 g or 12 tps of sugar from all sources per day. Ideally our sugar consumption should be no more than half this amount.

How Do You Know if You Are Addicted to Sugar?

If you answer yes to any of the following questions then you are likely to have a level of addiction to sugar.

- Do you have routines around sugar consumption such as buying a chocolate bar most nights on the way home from work?
- Do you need sugar hits daily?
- If forced to go without sugar for 24 hours, do you develop headaches and mood swings?
- Do you struggle to walk past a sugary treat without having 'just one'?

eat a rainbow a day

Most of us realise we need to eat more fruit and vegetables. What we may not realise is that we also need to eat a variety of different-coloured fruits and vegetables daily. Different coloured fruits and vegetables have different nutrients and so variety in our diet is essential for us to get all that our body needs from these foods. Simply eating the same piece of fruit each day and just lettuce on our sandwich does not cut it. Ideally we need to aim to eat a rainbow a day of coloured fruits and vegetables. That is, we need to consume all seven colours of the fruit and vegetable rainbow every day to receive the protection we need from chronic diseases.

Health TIP

Enjoying a variety of different-coloured fruits and vegetables ensures we are getting enough of the necessary micronutrients from our food.

People who eat a variety of different coloured fruits and vegetables as part of a healthy diet have reduced risk of chronic diseases including stroke, type 2 diabetes, some types of cancer, heart disease and high blood pressure[1]. This is because fruits and vegetables are coloured differently due to the presence of different phytonutrients, which are powerful antioxidants. Below is a list of the different colours that we find in fruit and vegetables and what this means in terms of different nutrients.

Eating a Rainbow a Day Keeps the Doctor Away

ORANGE FRUITS & VEGETABLES

These are usually coloured by natural plant pigments called 'carotenoids'. Beta-carotene in sweet potatoes, pumpkins and carrots is converted to vitamin A, which helps maintain healthy mucous membranes and healthy eyes. Scientists have also reported that carotenoid-rich foods can help reduce the risk of cancer and heart disease and can improve immune system function[1].

Some examples of the orange group include:

- Carrots
- Apricots
- Squash
- Cantaloupe
- Pumpkin
- Sweet potatoes
- Mangoes
- Sweet corn
- Papayas

RED FRUITS AND VEGETABLES

These are coloured by natural plant pigments called 'lycopene' or 'anthocyanins'. Lycopene in tomatoes, watermelon and pink grapefruit, for example, may help reduce the risk of several types of cancer, especially prostate cancer[2]. Lycopene in foods containing cooked tomatoes, such as spaghetti sauce and a small amount of fat are absorbed better than lycopene from raw tomatoes. Anthocyanins in strawberries, raspberries, red grapes and other fruits and vegetables act as powerful antioxidants that protect cells from damage.

These are some examples of the red group:

- Red apples
- Beets
- Red cabbage
- Cherries
- Cranberries
- Pink grapefruit
- Red grapes
- Tomatoes
- Red capsicum (peppers)
- Pomegranates
- Red potatoes
- Radishes
- Raspberries
- Rhubarb
- Strawberries
- Watermelon

YELLOW/ORANGE FRUITS & VEGETABLES

Citrus fruits like oranges, tangerines, lemons, limes and grapefruit are an excellent source of vitamin C and citrus bioflavonoids. Citrus bioflavonoids are a powerful antioxidant that prevents allergies and inflammation and may prevent bruising, haemorrhoids, varicose veins and spider veins[3].

These are some examples of the yellow/orange group include:

- Oranges
- Lemons
- Limes
- Yellow grapefruit
- Tangerines/mandarins

RED/PURPLE FRUITS & VEGETABLES

These are coloured by anthocyanins (see above). Anthocyanins in blueberries, grapes and raisins act as powerful antioxidants that protect cells from damage. They may also help reduce risk of cancer, stroke and heart disease. Other studies have shown that eating more blueberries is linked to improved memory function and healthy ageing[4].

These are some examples of the red/purple group:

- Blackberries
- Blueberries
- Eggplant
- Figs
- Raspberries
- Purple grapes
- Raisins
- Prunes
- Plums
- Red cabbage

YELLOW/GREEN FRUITS & VEGETABLES

These are coloured by a natural plant pigment called 'chlorophyll'. Some members of the green group, including spinach and other dark leafy greens, green peppers, peas, cucumber and celery, contain lutein. Lutein works with another chemical, zeaxanthin, found in corn, red peppers, oranges, grapes and egg yolks, to help keep eyes healthy. Together, these chemicals may help reduce the risk of cataracts and age-related macular degeneration[5], which can lead to blindness if untreated. Leafy greens such as spinach and broccoli are excellent sources of folate, a B vitamin that helps reduce the risk of birth defects.

Some examples of the yellow-green group include:

- Green apples
- Artichokes
- Asparagus
- Avocados
- Green beans
- Broccoli
- Brussels sprouts
- Honeydew melon
- Kiwi
- Lettuce
- Limes
- Green onions
- Peas
- Green grapes
- Green cabbage
- Spinach
- Green pepper
- Cucumbers
- Zucchini

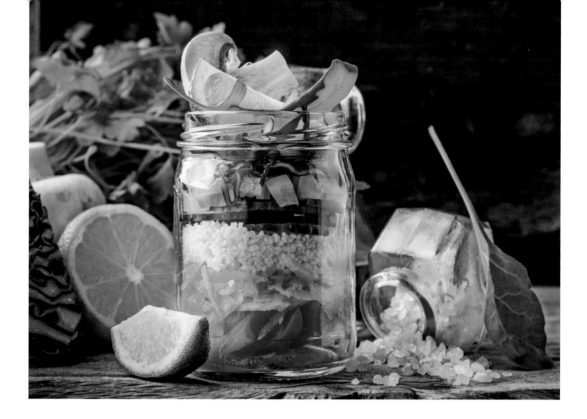

GREEN VEGETABLES

The 'indoles' in the cruciferous vegetables, such as broccoli, cauliflower, cabbage and brussels sprouts, may help protect against some types of cancer including breast, prostate and colon cancer[6].

Examples of green vegetables include:

- Broccoli
- Brussels sprouts
- Cabbage
- Cauliflower

WHITE FRUITS AND VEGETABLES

These are coloured by anthoxanthins (see above). They contain health-promoting chemicals such as allicin, which may help lower cholesterol and blood pressure and may help reduce the risk of stomach cancer and heart disease[1]. Some members of the white group, such as bananas and potatoes, are also good sources of the mineral potassium.

Some examples of the white group include:

- Bananas
- Onions
- Cauliflower
- Parsnips
- Garlic
- Potatoes
- Ginger
- Turnips
- Mushrooms

Ideally when it comes to fruit-and-vegetable intake we should be aiming to eat at least 5 serves of vegetables per day and around 2 serves of fruit per day. Many people eat adequate amounts of fruit but not enough vegetables. Some suggestions for increasing vegetable intake would be to eat a large salad for lunch every day, have a stir-fry for dinner, or even hide vegetables in casseroles, bolognaise, lasagnes etc. I even have a patient who includes vegetables like spinach, kale and carrot in homemade muffins and adds cocoa powder to disguise the taste.

If you find that you consistently are missing out on eating, or are even avoiding, a certain group of fruit and/or vegetables consider taking a powdered supplement. These can come as a general fruit/vegetable extract containing concentrated phytonutrients or as a specific coloured powder, usually green, which contains concentrated nutrients from that specific group. Eating the whole fruit or vegetable is always going to be more beneficial but adding a powdered supplement is an acceptable trade-off if you or your child simply cannot stand to eat fruit or vegetables.

Take Home Points

Different coloured fruits and vegetables contain different phytonutrients, which are powerful antioxidants that help protect us against cancer, heart disease, strokes, diabetes and other chronic diseases.

- Many of us do not eat enough different coloured fruits and vegetables and therefore are likely to be missing out on the different beneficial nutrients found in these.
- The seven different colours of fruits and vegetables make up the so-called phytonutrient rainbow.
- Try and aim to eat a fruit or vegetable from each of the phytonutrient rainbow colours per day.
- Tips for including more fruits and/or vegetables in your diet include eating a large salad for lunch, a stir-fry for dinner, adding plenty of vegetables to baked dishes, and even hiding them in casseroles, bolognaise and even in muffins.

YOUR *Weekly* CHALLENGE . . . .

This week your challenge is to eat a rainbow of different coloured fruits and vegetables every day. Choose, for example, to eat a large salad every day for lunch this week as an easy way to eat the majority of these in one sitting.

eat with the seasons

Mother Nature is wonderfully intuitive. She provides what we need in terms of nutrition all year round. In fact, she is so intuitive she provides certain fruits and vegetables at particular times of the year just when we need them in higher amounts.

With the modernisation of the way we purchase and cultivate produce it is difficult to know which fruits and vegetables are actually in season. Produce can be grown on the other side of the world, picked whilst still green and then ripened artificially with ethylene gas. So what we see on the supermarket shelves is not always what we would find growing locally at that particular time of year. I am often surprised to see that no matter where I go in the world supermarket shelves are filled with produce transported to places far away from the country of origin - oranges grown in California sold in Australia and mangoes grown in Australia sold in California.

What Are the Benefits of Eating Seasonal Produce?

Locally grown fruits and vegetables are thought to be higher in mineral and vitamin content due to not being harvested before they have matured and absorbing their full nutrient quota from the soil[1,2]. Also, the mineral and vitamin content of this produce is intended to match the needs of consumers living in the same area as the produce itself[1,2]. This is a type of process in nature called symbiosis; a term I loosely define as harmony in living.

Health FACT . . . .

Eating seasonally benefits our health and the environment, and supports local farmers.

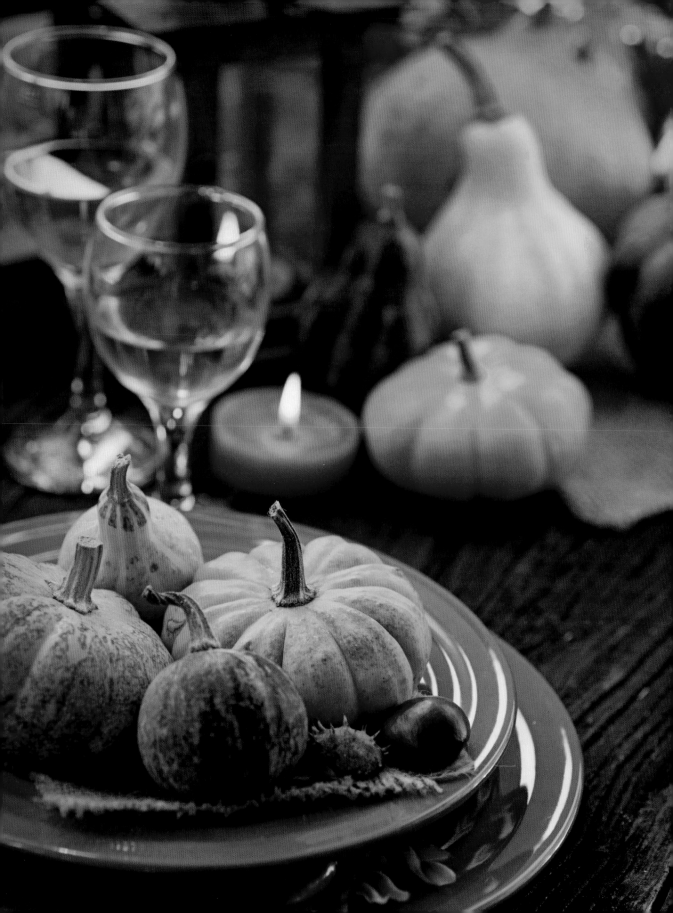

Take oranges, for example, which are rich in vitamin C, needed for our immune system[3]. Oranges are principally ripe during the winter months[4]. These are times when respiratory and other viruses are at their peak and our bodies require a greater intake of vitamin C to fight these assailants. Another example is spinach and kale, which are rich in zinc[3], another immune-booster in its own right. These dark, leafy vegetables are also found in winter[4]. In summer, we require a greater intake of water, natural sugar and electrolytes, which are principally found in summer fruits such as watermelon, grapes, cantaloupe, mangoes, and pineapple[3,4]. This is also the case with salad vegetables which have a high water content, making them the perfect summer-meal companion.

Not only is eating seasonally better for your health and the health of the environment (due to a reduction in transportation greenhouse emissions), but it supports local farmers and often is cheaper as a result. Compare, for instance, the cost of produce on your supermarket shelves that is out of season, which has often been transported from across the world, refrigerated and stored only partially ripened. The cost for storage and transportation is quite high compared with fruit and vegetables from your local farmer's market, where the produce is often fresher and richer in flavour, not to mention rich in vitamins and minerals.

To buy seasonally, however, requires a shift in our assumption that the same produce will be available all year long. Our recipes need to adapt as produce-availability changes. For a list of seasonal recipes visit Better Health Channel[5].

It is actually quite a treat to look forward to the taste of the new fruits and vegetables available in the coming season, much like Grandma would have experienced. I recall a Russian patient of mine who grew up in times where food was scarce telling the story of how the children in her town were delighted to see the fruit truck arrive with fresh oranges in winter. This was looked forward to more than chocolate or other treat.

How Do You Eat Seasonally?

Firstly, look for farmers' markets in your local area. These aren't hard to find and are usually listed in the local newspaper. If you are unable to find a farmer's market, choose to purchase mainly seasonal produce at your supermarket, which is often the produce that is the cheapest and is usually on special. A list of seasonal produce available in Australia can also be found by referring to seasonalfoodguide.com.

Try growing your own vegetables and fruits. Even just growing some basic herbs, tomatoes, strawberries and chillies, for example, can save on the food bill and ensure you have fresh produce readily available. Joining a community co-op garden can be a good way to share produce as well as build connections with like-minded individuals.

Finally, and this is the cherry on the top, attempt to purchase organic fruits and vegetables. These are grown without harmful chemicals and pesticides and are cultivated in soils rich in nutrients that the produce, and in turn our bodies, require[6]. Commercially cultivated produce has been shown to be grown in poorer soil quality[6]. Whilst of course this depends on your budget, I certainly feel that it would be a wise investment. Even choosing to purchase organic fruits and vegetables that do not contain a thick peel is a great start e.g. spinach, lettuce, tomato, broccoli, cabbage etc. At least with produce that has a thick peel you can reduce the chemical and pesticide load in your body by throwing out the peel e.g. bananas, oranges, and watermelon.

With all that said, I think if we would attempt to purchase seasonal produce a little more often and support our local farmers we would undoubtedly make Mother Nature proud. Ultimately, this is living the way things were intended.

Take Home Points

Eating seasonally is the way Mother Nature intended.

- We require higher amounts of different nutrients at different times of the year and these different nutrients are found in the amounts we need in the seasonally available produce.
- Often, produce that is not seasonal is grown overseas and then needs to be refrigerated only partially ripened, often waxed to protect it, sometimes irradiated, and then transported sometimes thousands of kilometres away.
- Produce that is grown locally is often higher in nutrient content, is cheaper, and is readily available.
- Adapt your recipes to whatever produce is seasonally available.
- Consider growing your own produce, even if this is just herbs and a few small vegetables.
- Other sources of seasonal produce are local farmers markets and community co-op gardens, which also promote rich community integration and interaction.

YOUR *Weekly* CHALLENGE . . . .

This week your challenge is to buy local seasonal produce and therefore benefit your health, save money and help out your local farmers. Check out your local farmer's market this week and also consider investing in organic produce where you can afford it.

eat out with confidence

Eating out is more and more common as our lives have become busier. The problem with this is that so many foods that we are able to buy in cafés and restaurants are not that good for us. Knowing which ones are better choices might make all the difference when it comes to being able to stick to our healthy eating plan. This is especially the case if we are in a foreign town or country and we find ourselves having to buy food at a local eatery. Abiding by some simple principles when it comes to eating out means we can make choices with the confidence that we are not undoing all our hard work. Before we look at what these principles might be, let us briefly examine why takeaway foods can be so bad for us.

Health FACT . . . .

You can still eat healthily when you choose to eat out as long as you stick to a few simple guidelines.

Avoid the Peril of MSG

MSG is short for monosodium glutamate. It is a flavour enhancer that is added to some takeaway foods to improve the taste. In essence MSG tricks your brain into thinking the food tastes good by stimulating your taste buds. It also stimulates your appetite and can trigger an addiction to that food to which MSG has been added. It looks similar to salt and mixes in with the food like salt so you will not realise that it is present.

Most commonly MSG is found added to Asian-style foods – Chinese, Korean and Thai takeaway foods. Keep in mind that MSG can also be found naturally in a lot of foods, including meats, diary products, tomatoes, soy products, nuts and beans, as the natural chemical glutamate, which is metabolised into MSG in the body. The problem is that the amount artificially added to some takeaway foods is very high, much more than would normally be found in foods naturally.

In some individuals who are MSG sensitive the body reacts badly when they ingest it. Symptoms that occur within an hour of eating a food containing MSG and can include:

- Dry mouth
- Stomach cramps
- Nausea/vomiting
- Diarrhoea
- Migraine headaches
- Heart palpitations
- Rapid heartbeat
- Shortness of breath
- Light-headedness
- Joint pain/stiffness
- Blurry vision

Other conditions have also recently been linked to MSG[1] including:

Obesity MSG may damage a part of the brain that regulates appetite called the 'hypothalamus'. A damaged hypothalamus may lead to a runaway appetite and therefore potential weight gain. MSG has also been found to trigger the pancreas to produce more insulin, which in turn reduces blood sugar. This is why many people are hungry an hour or so after eating food containing MSG.

Excitotoxicity Research has shown that MSG can cause lesions in the brain by killing off brain cells by literally exciting them to death. The young are most susceptible and so keep MSG foods away from children.

Keep in mind that MSG can also be found in processed foods such as some salad dressings, gravies, soups, stocks, soy sauce and processed meats. It is often renamed on the ingredients list as hydrolysed vegetable or plant protein, yeast extract, soy protein isolate, natural flavours or as enhancer 621. So to avoid MSG always ask at Asian-style restaurants if their food is MSG-free. Read labels well when you are at the supermarket and where possible avoid processed foods as this will reduce the chance that you are unknowingly ingesting MSG.

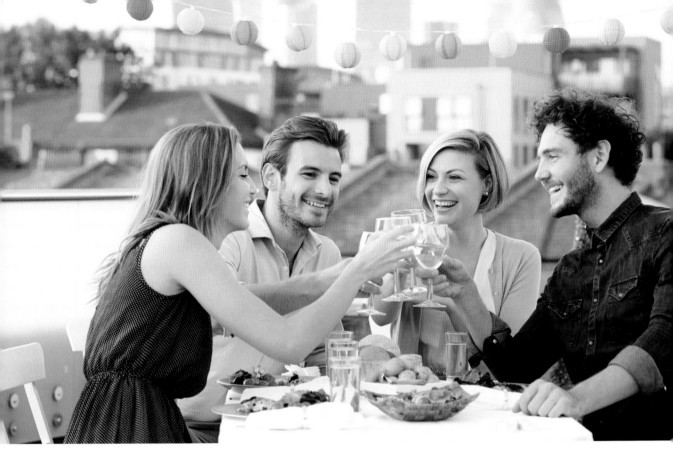

The Tasty Triplet - Fat, Sugar & Salt

Often takeaway foods are much higher in fat, sugar and salt content than home-cooked food. This is obviously intended to enhance the flavour of foods to increase their palatability and tempt you to buy the food again. The other problem comes with the type of fat used for cooking. Often cheap hydrogenated vegetable oil is used for cooking and frying. Fat that has been hydrogenated is linked to heart disease and should be avoided. So how do we avoid this tasty triplet, as well as MSG, if we are buying out?

Tips for How You Can Eat Out With Confidence

Making healthy choices when eating out at restaurants and cafes can be tricky, but with these simple tips we can choose better options.

HEALTHIER BREAKFAST TAKEAWAYS

- Avoid pre-prepared juices. These contain so much hidden sugar and are not the healthy choice we think they are. If you really feel like a juice, ask for a freshly prepared vegetable juice with only one piece of fruit such as a green apple to add some sweetness. Alternatively, opt for a berry smoothie instead as these are lower in glycaemic index than a juice.

- Choose poached or boiled eggs instead of fried. Add a side serve of grilled tomato, spinach, mushrooms and asparagus. If eating bread, stick to one slice and opt for multigrain, rye or spelt.
- Fresh fruit with yoghurt is also a good option.
- Choose one piece of raisin toast rather than two.
- Bircher muesli is packed full of nutrients but is very energy dense so keep your serving size small.
- Avoid pancakes and French toast.

HEALTHIER LUNCH TAKEAWAYS

- Choose salad options with protein such as grilled chicken salad.
- Keep dressings on the side rather than pre-mixed.
- Choose salads without cheese, like garden salad.
- Steer away from deep-fried options.
- Steer away from a lot of bread including white gluten-free. Choose a wrap instead. If eating a sandwich ask for an open sandwich instead, or just eat one slice of bread rather than both. Choose lean cuts of meat such as turkey or ham, or tuna or salmon as filling options. Opt for as much salad as possible and choose avocado instead of mayonnaise or margarine.
- If choosing Japanese, for example sushi, opt for brown rice sushi and stick to grilled chicken, avocado, tuna, salmon, and vegetarian options. Steer away from teppanyaki and deep-fried. The best option is sashimi with or without a small serve of brown rice.
- Vietnamese rice paper rolls or clear noodle soup is a good option.
- Choose water or green tea as a drink.
- Avoid soft drinks, juice, smoothies, iced teas and cordial.

HEALTHIER DINNER TAKEAWAYS

Mediterranean Avoid the bread. One medium bread roll can be equal to the same amount of calories as a palm-sized piece of meat or chicken. You can either choose the bread or the meat but not both – I know what I would rather have! Avoid main meal sizes and instead choose entrée sizes for meals. If having pasta, opt for tomato based instead of carbonara or cream sauces. Choose grilled fish, chicken or lamb with garden salad and dressing on the side. Share a dessert – the best option being sorbet with fruit. Avoid pizza.

Asian Choose clear soups such as miso and rice-noodle soups. Opt for stir-fries rather than deep fried dishes. Avoid curries, coconut-milk based meals and skip the entrée and go straight to a main meal.

Stick to 1-2 glasses of wine or beer. Choose mineral water with lemon or lime if you still feel like something 'special' to drink.

As with anything, moderation is the key. If you keep your serving size small then you can enjoy your meal and be a little less selective with what you choose. Keep in mind that if you only eat out infrequently then choose any option you feel like but remember to get back onto your healthy eating plan the following day.

Take Home Points

- More and more we are eating out at cafés and restaurants.
- Takeaway and restaurant foods can be high in salt, sugar and fats and may have added MSG.
- It is also very easy to eat more than you usually would due to larger serving sizes.
- Healthier takeaway breakfast options include fresh fruit, plain Greek yoghurt, poached or boiled eggs, grilled tomato, spinach and mushrooms. Muesli in small amounts is also a healthy option. Choose multigrain breads, rye or spelt rather than white breads, wholemeal or white gluten-free bread.
- Healthier takeaway lunch options include salad with grilled meat, chicken or fish. Clear soups, wraps, and brown-rice sushi rolls are healthier options. Avoid deep fried takeaway foods. Choose water and green tea as drinks rather than soft drinks, juice, iced teas and flavoured milk.
- Healthier takeaway dinner options include clear soups, thinner crust pizzas with lighter toppings, pasta with tomato-based sauces and grilled fish with salad. Steer away from bread rolls and choose entrée-sized main meals. Ask for a side serve of steamed vegetables or garden salad if you think you will still be hungry.

YOUR *Weekly* CHALLENGE . . . .

This week your aim is to make wise choices when you are buying meals out. By choosing healthier options for breakfast, lunch and/or dinner when you are buying at a café or restaurant you will still be able to stick to your healthy eating plan and not feel guilty.

buy smart & don't spend a fortune

I have heard it said that eating healthily can be expensive. And holding on to this notion can prevent people from leading a healthy lifestyle. Although I realise that the cost of living in general has increased over recent years I do not feel that living a healthy lifestyle needs to place us under financial strain. There are some clever ways to buy good food without the expense; we just need to know where to shop and what to buy. Some items in our pantry are worth spending extra money on, and others we can get without breaking the bank. The flipside is that I believe that every dollar we spend on living a healthy lifestyle and eating well is money well spent; especially when you compare the personal cost of being unhealthy versus being healthy. Let us briefly examine the personal cost of being unhealthy and then look at ways we can save each week on our food bill.

What Is The Cost of Living Healthily Vs Unhealthily?

A recent study from the *British Medical Journal* (BMJ) shows that it only has to cost an extra A$1.66 a day to eat healthy food as opposed to unhealthy food[1]. That makes it A$606 dearer a year to eat healthily compared to eating less healthy foods like those high in saturated fats and sugars and refined carbohydrates. This isn't even the cost of a cup of coffee a day and hardly seems like a significant amount of money given the burdens associated with being unhealthy. The pinnacle of which are the health costs associated with obesity.

Health FACT . . . .

Studies have shown that it only costs on average $1.66 more a day to eat healthily as opposed to unhealthily[1].

The level of obesity is the highest it has ever been in Australia and it's on the rise. Around ¼ of adult Australians are currently obese[2]. This level is expected to peak at over 80 per cent of Australians and ⅓ of children by 2025[2]. Obesity is expensive and costs society and individuals money that we simply do not have to spend.

The Preventative Health Taskforce paper on obesity illustrates the impact of this condition on overall health and the health-care system. The report shows that the burden of disease attributable solely to high body mass is now close to that of smoking[3]. Obesity has been directly linked to about ¼ of type 2 diabetes (23.8 per cent) and osteoarthritis (24.5 per cent), ⅕ of cardiovascular disease (21.3 per cent) and colorectal, breast, uterine and kidney cancers (20.5 per cent)[3]. Obesity puts an enormous strain on the country's economy.

In 2008 it was estimated that the overall worldwide cost of obesity to society and governments was $58.2 billion[3]. Individually, a study published in the *Medical Journal of Australia* in 2010 revealed that the annual total direct cost (health-care and non-health-care) per person increased from $1472 per year for those of normal weight to $2788 for those who are obese[4]. That's an extra cost of around $1300 a year. With these costs in mind it certainly seems like it pays to lead a healthy lifestyle. As food is often one of the largest expenses in our budget, how then do we save on the cost of eating?

	UNHEALTHY PERSON	HEALTHY PERSON	DIFFERENCE BETWEEN UNHEALTHY & HEALTHY
Average Estimated Lifetime Food Cost[5]	$365 000	$400 000	$35 000 more to eat healthy per lifetime
Average Life Expectancy[5]	80	84	Life expectancy reduced by 4 years
Susceptible Diseases[3]	Heart disease, type 2 diabetes, obesity, cancers and depression	Reduced risk of these diseases. Increased protection towards bowel, breast cancer	Increased risk of chronic diseases
Average Personal Cost of Health-care per Annum[4]	$1669 for overweight; $2788 for obese	$1472 per annum for person of healthy weight	Between $197–$1306 more per annum on health-care
Average Government Expenditure on Health-care per Annum[4]	$21 billion for overweight and obese	$10.3 billion for person of normal weight	$10.7 billion more government expense

How You Can Eat Healthily on a Budget

The cost of buying healthy foods can add up if you are not aware of the huge variation in health-food prices. Below are my top ten tips for eating healthy on a budget.

Tip # 1 Avoid Processed Foods Food items labelled as 'health foods' can be expensive and may not actually be that good for you. An example of this is gluten-free foods – many of which are refined white foods. The cost of foods that are processed and packaged can quickly add up. Avoiding products that are in packets and instead making your own can save big dollars. Remember to stick to the perimeter of the supermarket as much as possible, which is where the healthier, unprocessed foods, and often less expensive items, are kept.

Tip #2 Shop Smart The best healthy foods out there are the humble fruit and veg. Shop around and find the best deal. Visit your local greengrocer or local farmers' market and buy frozen items if needed to save on the cost of fresh e.g. frozen berries.

Tip #3 Buy in Bulk Buying essential items in bulk can definitely save on cost e.g. nuts, rice, beans, rolled oats. Look around for specials and stock up on pantry staples e.g. beans, tinned fruit etc.

Tip #4 Know What to Spend Money On It is worth spending money on fresh produce. Consider spending a little more for organic or at least chemical-spray free produce. Certain fruit and vegetables retain a higher pesticide load and my suggestion would be to choose these as organic/spray free. These include broccoli, spinach, berries and lettuce. Other items where spending a few extra dollars is worth it are with hormone-free poultry and meat. Choosing fresh fish rather than frozen will ensure the best quality and nutrient value. Establishing a good relationship with your local butcher and fishmonger is well worth the effort for the freshest and tastiest meat.

Tip # 5 Pack Your Lunch This simple step can save you literally thousands of dollars per year, especially if you are buying lunch out daily. Packing your lunch requires a little planning and time but will also improve your health.

Tip #6 Buy a Coffee Machine Many people buy at least 1 coffee a day. It is not uncommon for people to spend up to 20 or even 30 dollars per week on café bought coffee. This can, once again, equate to over 1000 dollars per year spent on coffee. My suggestion would be saving the trip to the café to special occasions such as meeting up with friends, or at least consider alternating days where one day you make yourself a coffee and the alternate day you buy a coffee.

Tip #7 Carry Snacks Being caught out hungry without a snack means you are going to be tempted to buy a snack. These are often overpriced and full of sugar, salt and/

or fat. Inexpensive snacks that keep fresh include fruit, nuts, homemade biscuits, rice crackers, or vegetables such as snow peas, cherry tomatoes, celery and carrots.

Tip # 8 Buy a Slow Cooker A slow cooker or similar device not only saves time but can mean that a meal is ready to eat when you get home from work. This makes the temptation to stop on the way home and spend money on takeaway food less likely.

Tip #9 Consider a Co-Op Consider finding or even establishing in your local area a food co-op. This is where you purchase items wholesale in bulk and share between several people to save on costs. There is bound to be a co-op in your community. It's also a great way to meet other like-minded healthy people.

Tip #10 Grow Your Own Growing your own produce can save on costs too. There are many ways to do this, from herb gardens to full-scale vegie patches. Even if you live in an apartment there are clever, space-saving ways to grow produce on your balcony. Some cities also have local community gardens where organic produce is grown and shared between community members for a small membership fee.

With these simple steps we can all be healthy without blowing the budget. It just requires a little planning and knowing how to buy smart.

Take Home Points

It is a myth that eating healthily is a lot more expensive than not eating healthily. Studies have shown that it only costs, on average, less than a cup of coffee per day to eat healthier.

- Eating healthily actually saves us money long-term in terms of health expenditure.
- Top tips to saving on the cost of eating include buying local, fresh produce, avoiding packaged foods and buying in bulk. Growing your own produce, joining a co-op and packing your lunches is also a great way to save big dollars on your food bill.
- Small changes and adjustments to our buying practices add up to big savings on our grocery bill each week.

YOUR *Weekly* CHALLENGE . . . .

This week your challenge is to save on your grocery bill by following some of the simple steps suggested in this chapter. Consider for example buying your produce from the local farmers market, buying in bulk, meeting your local butcher and/or fishmonger, and/or perhaps planting your own herbs this week.

plan well
plan to succeed

Planning really is the key to success when it comes to our health goals. Unfortunately just hoping one day we will have the time to get healthier will not happen. Life just seems to get busier and busier as we accumulate more responsibilities. So the only way to have the time to exercise, plan meals, stop and eat well and sleep well is to plan it into our schedules and vehemently protect our plan. There will be multiple factors that will attempt to threaten all our hard planning work but this is where the word 'No' comes in handy. We have to learn to be a little selfish in this regard and realise that 'I am the only person who can look after me and if I do not look after myself then I will not be able to look after anyone else'.

Health TIP

Planning our week helps to keep us focussed on our health goals.

I have seen so many men and women suffer poor health that just seemed to 'creep up on them'. In reality, life just passed them by and they forgot to plan into their schedules what should have been a priority to them. I suggest writing a weekly plan and sticking with it. Of course you can make adjustments to the plan as the need arises, but as a general guide the plan will help keep you on track. Post your weekly plan on the refrigerator - that way you will be reminded of it whenever you are tempted to forgo your health goals.

How to Plan Weekly

Keep in mind when you write a weekly plan that you need to allow margins in your schedule between appointments and activities so that you are not stressed out trying to get from one thing to the next. This creates unnecessary tension and takes the enjoyment out of life. Try to get to appointments 5-10 minutes early and practise deep breathing or meditation while you are waiting rather than checking emails on your mobile phone.

There are also several other elements to an effective plan:

Make time You have to make the time to write down your plan in advance. This will initially take about an hour. Your plan can then be reviewed monthly to see if it needs to be altered.

Keep it simple Keeping your plan as fuss-free as possible will help with being able to stick with it.

There is No Failure When it comes to making and sticking with your plan there will be times when you just will not be able to. That is okay and part of life. You have not 'failed', you just need to get back on track as soon as you are able to.

Co-ordinate schedules If you have a partner and/or dependent children you will need to consider their schedules as well. It surprises me how busy schooling and extra-curricular activities have become. It is not uncommon for me to hear Mums or Dads say that every afternoon and on the weekends their time is taken up with sporting and other activities. If you find yourself in this same situation consider that you probably only have two options: You either do everything yourself, including all the driving to and from activities and all the cooking and cleaning and forgo your own health goals, or you outsource and ask friends and family to help. You may organise, for instance, a car pool with another family, hire a cleaner, or even just ask your mum or trusted neighbour to mind the kids while you go for a jog around the block.

Jacqui's Weekly Plan

Meet Jacqui - she is a single, working woman in her early thirties. She works full-time and has decided to make a weekly plan to feel healthy again. Her weekly plan could look something like this:

DAY/TIME	SUN	MON	TUES	WED	THURS	FRI	SAT
6:00	Sleep in	Wake	Wake	Wake	Wake	Wake	Wake
7:00	Sleep in	Brisk walk 40 min	Pilates class 40 min	Gym 50 min	Brisk walk 40 min	Rest day from exercise	Meditation 30 min
8:00	Sleep in	Breakfast Get ready for work	Breakfast Get ready for work	Breakfast Get ready for work	Breakfast Get ready for work	Breakfast Get ready for work	Gym 30 min
9:00	Bike ride 45 min	Work	Work	Work	Work	Work	R&R
10:00	Brunch	Snack	Snack	Snack	Snack	Snack	Brunch
11:00	R&R	Work	Work	Work	Work	Work	R&R
12:00	Light Lunch	Lunch	Lunch	Lunch	Lunch	Lunch	Light Lunch
1:00	Meal Plan	Work	Work	Work	Work	Work	R&R
2:00	Groceries	Work	Work	Work	Work	Work	R&R
3:00	Snack	Snack	Snack	Snack	Snack	Snack	Snack
4:00	R&R	Work	Work	Work	Work	Work	R&R
5:00	R&R	Work	Work	Work	Work	Work	Weekly goal setting
6:00	R&R	Yoga Class	TV	Groceries	TV	TV	R&R
7:00	Cook + Dinner	Cook + Dinner	Cook + Dinner	Cook + Dinner	Cook + Dinner	Out to Dinner	Cook + Dinner
8:00	Prepare lunch	Prepare lunch	Prepare lunch	Prepare lunch	Prepare lunch	Out to Dinner	R&R
9:00	Wind-down	Wind-down	Wind-down	Wind-down	Wind-down	Wind-down	Wind-down
10:00	Sleep	Sleep	Sleep	Sleep	Sleep	Sleep	Sleep

Looking at this plan there are several coloured items. These items I call the 'gold star' activities. These activities will help to improve Jacqui's overall health and wellbeing and are the priority items in her case.

Rest & Sleep (purple) Prioritising enough time to wind down and sleep is important for our overall mental and physical well-being. Rest and relaxation is just as important and needs to be factored into our schedules, even if it is just $\frac{1}{2}$ an hour per day or on the weekends.

Exercise (blue) Incorporating some aerobic ('huffy puffy'), resistance (weight-bearing), and stretching-type exercise throughout the week provides a great balance and helps to ensure that our bodies do not become susceptible to injury. Remember that the idea is to slowly build up how much you do and that some exercise is better than none.

Time for Meals (red) So many of us eat standing up or at our desk. Rather, make the time to stop all other activities and just concentrate on your meal. This helps with digestion and gives your mind a much needed mental pause.

Meal Planning & Shopping (green) Meal planning takes around 30 minutes once a week. Once the meal plan is done, shopping becomes easier. Buying produce several times per week helps to ensure you are eating good-quality fresh fruit and vegetables.

Goal Planning (pink) Once per week review how you felt your week went. Did you achieve your health goals. Is there anything that you would like to do differently etc.? Planning your health (and work/life) goals for the week ahead helps you to move forward and stay on track.

Take Home Points

Plan your weekly set-up to reach your health goals.

- Planning helps us to prioritise what activities are most important to us and helps to keep us on track.
- Items to include in your weekly plan include sleep and rest, exercise, meal planning, food shopping and goal setting.
- Try to leave margins in your schedule to give you plenty of time to get to appointments and to allow for activities that end up taking more time than expected.

YOUR *Weekly* CHALLENGE . . . .

This week your challenge is to write out a weekly plan. Attach it to your fridge and try to stick to it. Hereafter, review your plan weekly and make small adjustments as you need.

practise portion perfection

Portion control can be a challenge for all of us especially in today's society where food is aplenty. The average portion sizes have increased significantly over the last 30 years. Consider, for example, that in the 1980s the average coffee was sold in a Styrofoam cup and contained around 180 Calories. Now it is not uncommon for people to buy the largest sized coffee, which contains 3 times as much milk, caffeine and Calories. Without realising it, a slight increase in portion size can make a significant impact to your overall food intake and ultimately your waistline.

Health FACT

There is not one ratio of daily macronutrient proportions that is associated with good health but a range[1].

- ✓ 20–35 per cent fat
- ✓ 45–65 per cent carbohydrates
- ✓ 15–25 per cent protein

Even if you are eating well, too much of a good thing is still too much. Often when I do a food-and-diet assessment with a patient, on paper the types of foods they are eating all look very healthy. You could be left scratching your head wondering why, then, are they gaining weight. But on further assessment, when I have asked them to write down the size of their meals, snacks and drinks it is evident that their portion sizes have crept up and they are eating much more than they realise; albeit healthy kinds of foods. Most of us are eating way more than we really need to eat. Our body does not need a lot of fuel if we are feeding ourselves with nutritious options.

So what constitutes an appropriate portion size? The answer to this question is discussed below, along with tips on how to keep portion sizes down without feeling hungry or deprived.

How Much Is Enough?

The following list is a guide to what constitutes a portion for everyday foods[2].

- About a palm-sized serving of meat, chicken, tofu or fish for lunch and dinner
- 2 eggs is one serve. Allow 2 to 3 servings of eggs (or around 4–6 eggs) per week instead of another protein source
- Two serves of fruit per day (really no more than this unless you are particularly physically active as this adds extra natural sugar). Examples of a serve of fruit include $\frac{1}{2}$ large banana or mango, 2 small plums or apricots, a medium apple, pear, peach or nectarine, a small bunch of grapes or $\frac{1}{2}$ cup of cut melon
- Occasional fruit juice ($\frac{1}{2}$ glass) and dried fruit (around 30 g = $1\frac{1}{2}$ tbsp sultanas or 4 apricot halves) instead of 1 serving of fruit
- 2–3 cups of cooked vegetables or 4–5 cups of fresh salad per day
- 2–3 servings of dairy, which includes a matchbox-size of cheese (allow a maximum of 1–2 serves of cheese per day), a 250 mL glass of milk and/or 200 g of plain, unsweetened yoghurt per day
- A tennis-ball sized serve of rice, noodles, quinoa, polenta, oats or pasta (allow 1–2 serves per day)
- $\frac{1}{2}$ cup of cooked dried or canned lentils, peas or beans (if canned, choose varieties with no added salt)
- 2 slices of bread is 1 serve (allow 1–2 serves per day)
- A small bowl of cereal per day (around 1 cup depending on the cereal)
- A small handful of nuts per day (around 15 almonds, 10 brazil nuts, 15 cashews, 15 macadamia or a small handful of raw, unsalted mixed nuts)
- Two finger-widths size for the occasional snack such as a protein bar
- 1 tbsp of dressing or sauce with lunch or dinner
- 1 thin spread of butter or avocado on bread per day

For all other foods that constitute 'sometimes' foods – if you choose to eat these have in small amounts.

Tricks to Portion Control

The trick to portion control is to slightly alter your portion sizes so that you do not feel hungry or deprived. This extra amount that you would otherwise eat but not miss has been coined the 'mindless margin' and is easy enough to leave off your plates without noticing the difference. Up to 20 per cent of the food on our plate can easily be left off without making a noticeable difference to our hunger levels[3].

Some general tips to keeping portion sizes down include:

- Eat from smaller plates and bowls. Consider eating your main meal from an entrée-sized plate, and soups and desserts from a small children's-sized bowl rather than a large one. By eating from a smaller plate or bowl our brain is tricked into thinking we are eating the same amount of food because our meal still fills the entire plate/bowl.
- Fill at least half of your plate with salad or non-starchy vegetables (such as lettuce, spinach, broccoli, cauliflower, asparagus, squash, zucchini, eggplant, green beans). Since we make portion decisions with our eyes and not with our stomachs the trick is to fill your plate with these lower-calorie foods so that your brain still sees a full plate.
- $\frac{1}{4}$ of your plate can be topped with starches including rice, potatoes, corn, carrots, pasta, quinoa or noodles.
- $\frac{1}{4}$ can be a protein source, including meat, chicken, fish, tofu, lentils/beans.
- Drink from tall skinny glasses instead of short wide glasses as skinny glasses look fuller.
- Keep on hand small containers for portioning out snacks rather than eating from the original packaging.
- If making a large serving of a meal, portion-out into individual servings and freeze for another day/meal.
- Water down fruit juice or, better still, avoid completely and choose whole fruit instead (but avoid extra natural sugar).
- Choose a salad option when dining out (dressing on the side).
- Choose pre-packaged party-sized servings of chocolate and sweets to have as your occasional snack.
- Drink a large glass of water 10–15 minutes before a meal. This can curb appetite.
- Think 20 per cent less overall food on your plate and 20 per cent more vegetables or salad on your plate.

Hopefully with these simple tips we may all find managing our portions a little easier.

Take Home Points

Portion sizes have crept up, particularly in the last 2-3 decades.

- It has been noted that we can reduce our portions by 20 per cent without noticing a significant difference to how full we feel.
- Tricks to portion control include filling up your plate with plenty of low energy vegetables and salads.
- Include on your plate a serving of protein, which is typically a palm-sized serving of meat, chicken or fish.
- A serving of starch can also be added to your plate, which is typically a tennis-ball sized serving of rice, potatoes, sweet potato, carrot, peas, corn, pasta, quinoa or noodles.
- If you choose to add a dressing or sauce keep it to around a tbsp in size per meal.
- Drinking plenty of water throughout the day can also help to curb portion sizing.

YOUR *Weekly* CHALLENGE . . . .

This week your challenge is to reduce your portion sizes. Consider purchasing online a portion controlled plate and bowl as a guide of how much constitutes a healthy portion.

reduce mindless eating

A lot of the time we eat without even realising it. Whether it be eating an extra mouthful or two of our main meals past the point where we no longer feel hungry just because it is in front of us, or grabbing a handful of nuts from the cupboard while we are looking for something else just because we can. This all contributes significantly to our overall daily food intake. This type of eating pattern is called 'mindless eating' and means that we can eat way more than we want or plan to in a given day just because we are not aware of it. We are often focussing on something else at the time and so are completely oblivious to what we are putting in our mouths.

I have met patients who have for years struggled with their weight and when I ask them what they ate in the last 24 hours they often omit snack foods, whether it be a biscuit here or a piece of chocolate there. This often is not a conscious decision. They honestly just don't realise how many small snacks they were consuming throughout the day alongside their main meals. When I then ask them to write a food diary they are often shocked to discover that they actually eat a lot more than they realise. It is very easy for any one of us to do this as food is so abundantly present these days.

So how do you know if you are eating mindlessly? There are some basic questions you can ask yourself to gauge the amount of mindless eating that you are doing throughout the day.

- Do you eat whilst driving?
- Do you eat whilst reading the paper, watching TV, or working on the computer?
- Do you eat whilst talking on the phone?
- Do you eat whilst standing up?
- Do you eat out of large packets rather than serving yourself a smaller portion in a bowl?

- Do you eat when you are stressed, bored, tired, lonely, frustrated, anxious, sad or angry?
- Do you eat when happy, excited or nervous?
- Do you think about your next meal when you have not even finished your current meal?
- Do you often finish a meal or snack you are not really enjoying just because it is in front of you?

If you answered yes to any of these questions chances are you do quite a bit of mindless eating throughout the day. Mindless eating can contribute to at least 20 per cent more food intake throughout the day. Overall this can mean an extra 10 kg of body fat a year. When you are focussing on other things whilst you are eating it can be very difficult to gauge when you are full and when to stop.

Health FACT . . . .

We make around 200 decisions about eating every day with 90 per cent of these decisions made without conscious thought[1].

Also by developing a habit of associating eating and another activity, such as eating and driving, you are more likely to continue to look for something to eat every time you get into the car. This then creates a difficult habit to break and often requires an intermediate step such as replacing eating with drinking water or herbal tea, for example, which might serve the purpose of helping to wean off the habit of chewing when you are doing other activities.

How to Overcome Mindless Eating

It is important to at least be aware of when you are more likely to do mindless eating so that you can avoid eating more than your body needs and 'accidentally' putting on extra weight.

Some general tips to overcoming mindless eating include:

- Attempt to eat only at a designated place for meals such as the dining table or breakfast bar.
- Avoid eating on the couch, in bed or at your desk.
- Avoid eating whilst watching TV, working on the computer, reading or on the phone.
- Avoid eating whilst driving.

listen to your hunger cues

Hunger is a normal physiological drive to eat. If we ignore our hunger cues we will get to the point of feeling overwhelmingly ravenous. When this happens we step into survival mode and can be prone to making the wrong food choices. On the contrary, I have met people who have ignored their hunger cues for so long they no longer are aware of when they are truly hungry or whether they are eating out of appetite, which I will explain. There is a keen difference between hunger and appetite. Hunger will lead us to eat only when our body needs sustenance, whereas appetite drives us to eat out of an emotional need. We will discuss more about appetite, emotional eating and cravings in the next chapter, but for now let us take a look at what causes us to feel hungry and how we can learn to listen to our hunger cues as a way to avoid overeating and eating less healthy food.

Health FACT . . . .

Hunger is normal but many of us have lost touch with our body's hunger cues so that we swing between being ravenous and overfull.

Why Do We Get Hungry?

It is not uncommon for me to hear patients describe how they can go the whole day without eating due to being busy with work schedules and other tasks, but then as soon as they get home they realise how hungry they actually are. This often leads to high-hurdling the kitchen bench to get to the fridge and spending the next 20 minutes eating a large amount of food as quickly as possible in order to raise their blood sugar levels. This feeding frenzy is usually followed by skipping dinner, the very meal that has the most vegetable intake for most people These individuals, night after night, are missing out on eating the recommended serves of vegetables. Sooner or later they find they are carrying too much weight around their middles and not really realising that it has to do with this after-work eating pattern.

See, when our blood sugar falls below a certain level the hunger centre in a part of our brain called 'the hypothalamus' is activated, which compels us to eat. The main foods you will desire will be carbohydrates and sugars to raise blood sugar the fastest. The hungrier you are the more your body will crave them. These foods also raise serotonin, which is a neurotransmitter associated with feelings of fullness and well-being. When we eat foods that raise the blood sugar our hunger centre is then switched off. Our hunger centre can also be switched off by hormones that are released by the stretching of our stomach and by the presence of fats and proteins in our meal.

It is important not to skip meals as you will end up being too hungry and this can lead to an overwhelming desire to binge on the less healthy food options. Such foods are often addictive by their very nature and therefore all tend to lack the proper ratio of carbohydrates, proteins, fats and fibre to ensure that the hunger centre is turned off for many hours. Instead, these foods are rapidly absorbed and spike both blood sugar and insulin levels – leading to a cycle of consumption and craving for the wrong types of foods. Over time, it becomes harder to break this cycle as insulin levels become chronically elevated, causing fluctuations in blood sugar. And if the cycle continues, it is possible to become insulin resistant so that adequate blood sugar is never able to enter the cells – including those in the hypothalamus – and turn off the hunger centre in the brain. The result is a ravenous appetite and eventually pre-diabetes or type 2 diabetes.

Some people are so hungry they end up consuming large amounts of food in one sitting very quickly. What they do not realise is that this can lead to stretching of the stomach over time, meaning that you will need to eat more and more food to feel full. A bariatric surgeon friend of mine once mentioned to me that he often operates on people whose stomachs are 4 or even 5 times larger than they should be due to years of being overexpanded. Luckily the stomach is a muscle and can shrink with eating smaller portions over time.

The other thing to keep in mind about the speed at which we eat is that it takes around 20 minutes for the message that we are full to be conveyed from our stomachs to our brains. So slowing down the speed at which we eat means that the hunger centre in our brain will be switched off when we have had an appropriate amount to eat and we are likely to not overeat.

How Can You Learn to Listen to Your Hunger Cues?

I have heard other experts describe a sliding scale for hunger as a way to get back in touch with listening to your hunger cues. This sliding scale ranges from 0 to 10. To avoid overeating, eat when you feel like you are at level 2 hunger and stop eating when you are at level 5 on the hunger scale i.e. when you are just full. This takes practice and involves getting back in touch with our physical hunger cues. Look out for signs of hunger such as foggy headedness, headaches, poor concentration, rumbling stomach and/or nausea.

Try not to allow yourself to get to level zero on the scale. This means you are likely to be ravenously hungry and have a higher chance of overeating. Recognise when you are starting to feel full and make a decision to take just a few more mouthfuls. Learn to dislike feeling overfull. I have a few patients who have yo-yo dieted for so many years that their mind convinces them that it is better to feel overfull in an attempt to prevent starvation. Once you stop yo-yo dieting you can once again experience the sensations of feeling a little hungry and then feeling appropriately satisfied by eating without feeling absolutely stuffed full.

Empty	Getting Empty	Full	Overfull	Stuffed
0	2	5	8	10

Tips to Managing Hunger

In order to manage the see-saw of hunger in a healthy way consider following these simple tips:

- Maintain a stable blood sugar level throughout the day by consuming regular, balanced meals and snacks (around every 3-3½ hours).
- Choose healthy, low GI foods that release sugar into the bloodstream slowly and therefore avoid sugar spikes and a runaway appetite as a result.
- Eat meals containing carbohydrates, proteins, fats and fibre as this helps you feel fuller for longer (protein, fat and fibre help slow down digestion) and avoids swings in blood sugar levels.
- Slow down your eating by chewing slowly and by chewing each mouthful around 20 times. Putting your fork down between bites and taking some deep breaths between bites can also be effective ways to slow eating. Take around 20 minutes to finish main meals as this is how long it takes for the message to reach your brain that you are full.
- Keep in mind the hunger sliding scale and aim to eat when feeling empty and stop when you are full.

- Before every meal ask yourself if you are really hungry or just eating because the clock says it is time to eat; or whether you are eating to soothe an emotion.
- Watch out for the first deep breath that you take towards the end of a meal as this is a sign that your body is satisfied and you should stop eating.

If we can manage our hunger better and avoid the massive swings in blood sugar that many people experience throughout the day we will be able to avoid overeating. This can help to curb appetite and cravings, minimise the possibility of gaining unwanted weight and developing diabetes, and help us to avoid the mood swings that can come with fluctuations in blood sugar.

Take Home Points

Hunger is a physiological drive to eat. It is normal to feel hungry and to want to curb that hunger with food.

- If we have allowed ourselves to get too hungry and then attempt to curb that hunger with excessive carbohydrates and sugar because we are ravenous, this can becomes an issue.
- Over time this can lead to an inability to properly gauge our hunger cues, weight gain, insulin resistance, and type 2 diabetes.
- To reset our hunger centre in the brain to detect appropriate levels of hunger and satisfaction from food, consider learning to listen to your hunger cues again.
- Learn to dislike feeling overfull and pace yourself when you eat to give your brain a chance to register that you are full.
- Observe when you take a deep breath towards the end of a meal as this is a subconscious signal your brain sends to let you know that you are full and to stop eating.

YOUR *Weekly* CHALLENGE . . . .

This week your challenge is to listen to your hunger cues and avoid allowing yourself to get too hungry or too full. Before every meal ask yourself if you are really hungry and then during a meal ask yourself if you are getting full.

overcome cravings

Cravings often arise because of our appetite. Appetite is different to hunger in that whilst hunger is a physiological need for food when our blood sugar levels fall, appetite is a psychological drive to satisfy an emotion or desire. In essence, appetite is hunger of the mind. You can have an appetite even when you know you are not hungry. This appetite is usually for foods or drinks that you crave as a way of emotional soothing. They are often sugary foods, carbohydrates, salty foods, caffeine or alcohol.

Health FACT

There is no pill that will overcome food cravings for you. Much of overcoming food cravings involves behavioural changes.

All these foods are therefore 'addictive' because they act as a form of analgesic, easing your stress or emotional pain. Because these types of foods release certain amounts of 'happy hormones' in your brain, as well as reset your tastebuds, they can

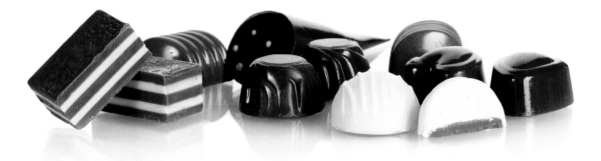

become addictive in their own right, too, as a food source. This means that you can start to crave them frequently and as you give in to this craving you will develop a habit of eating them at certain times of the day.

The struggle most people therefore have is not with hunger but with the appetite they have developed through years of poor dietary choices and as a coping strategy to overcome stress. A lot of people are no longer responding to true hunger but instead are attuned to satisfying their appetite.

As an aside, appetite can also be triggered by positive emotions, not just negative ones. Childhood memories associated with love, care, connection and food can be a trigger for some people. It is important therefore not to use food as a reward for children.

So although managing hunger involves purely physical solutions as we discussed in the previous chapter, cravings cannot be controlled without balancing brain chemistry.

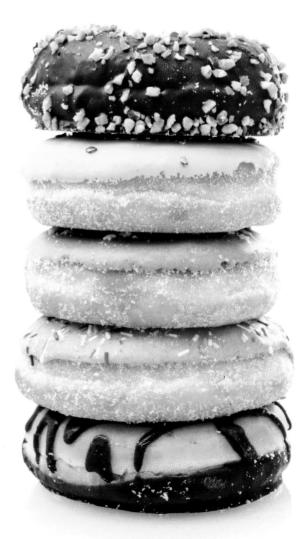

How to Overcome Your Cravings by Balancing Brain Chemistry

Brain chemistry involves three main brain chemicals that can lead to a runaway appetite – noradrenaline, serotonin and dopamine. These brain chemicals can become imbalanced because of stress, fatigue, anxiety, depression and, to some degree, our innate genetic tendencies and personality.

Noradrenaline deficiency This is our motivation brain chemical which is typically low in depression. It helps us to stay alert and focussed. When we are low in noradrenaline we can feel sluggish, tired, exhausted and have trouble concentrating. We will tend to binge-eat and crave starchy food.

Serotonin deficiency This is our feel-good brain chemical, which is typically low in depression and anxiety. Imbalance of this chemical is associated with sleep problems, cravings for sweets and carbohydrates especially in the afternoon and evening, binge eating, panic attacks, compulsive eating and mental fixation on foods. Interestingly, the female brain synthesises 50 per cent less serotonin than the male brain, which is thought to be the main reason why women crave sugars and starches more than men[1].

Dopamine deficiency This is our pleasure brain chemical. When you are low in dopamine you can become prone to developing addictions, including addictions to food. You will lack motivation, become irritable and moody and will crave caffeine to keep you going. You will likely have episodes of light-headedness, cloudy thinking and extreme hunger and will look for salty starchy foods like chips.

Aside from reducing stress levels and dealing with depression and anxiety through techniques mentioned in chapters to follow, supplements such as 5-hydroxytryptophan (5-HTP) can be used to raise serotonin levels and help control carbohydrate and sugar cravings. The typical dose is 100 mg 3 times per day on an empty stomach; although if you are taking anti-depressant medications do seek advice from your health-care practitioner before taking 5-HTP. Similarly the supplements L-tyrosine, S-adenosyl methionine, and N-acetyl L-tyrosine can be used to boost dopamine and noradrenaline levels, which helps to decrease appetite and cravings. The doses of these natural medications varies depending on the supplement so it is best to consult with your health-care practitioner before taking these.

Other Practical Strategies to Overcoming Your Food Cravings

There are a number of strategies that you may find helpful in overcoming food cravings including:

- Eat good quality foods every 3-3½ hours e.g. fruits and vegetables, proteins, and good fats contained in nuts, for example.

- Understand why and when you tend to crave foods (called 'trigger times') by writing a 4-day food diary - three weekdays and one weekend day. Write down your thoughts throughout the day around eating. The most common appetite trigger times are between 3-6pm and 8-11pm. Most people give in to these cravings and then will skip a meal to make up for it, which will set them up for another failure by lowering blood sugar to very low levels. It is important to maintain blood sugar levels by fuelling the body with the right type and amount of fuel i.e. a healthy breakfast, lunch and dinner with morning tea and afternoon tea and an evening snack if you eat dinner early.

- Keep water with you at all times as often the body confuses hunger with thirst. Take the edge off your craving by having a drink of water when you feel the desire to eat a less healthy option. Keep snacks handy that you can eat that will not only satisfy your hunger but also keep you on the right path towards healthy living.

- Alter your environment to remove tempting foods from your home, office, car etc. Do not keep these snacks in the house for your kids. You can choose to give them these snack foods once or twice a week outside of the home if you wish.

- Avoid mindless eating - eating when you are doing something else e.g. watching TV, on the computer. It only sets you up to eat more than you should and to associate the activity with food. The true pleasure of most foods is in the first few bites.

- Retrain your tastebuds. What you continually practise will eventually become a habit. Your body only wants what you normally give it. Retrain your tastebuds by not indulging in foods that are designed to get you hooked and learn to choose better options.

- Change your behaviour by being prepared for a craving when hunger sets in. You could try adopting the 'Five Ds' for when a craving sets in when you are not actually hungry i.e. emotional eating rather than hunger:

Delay Eating Avoid eating by 10-15mins (cravings come and go in waves).

Drink Water This can curb cravings.

Deep Breathe Take ten slow deep breaths to switch off the stress nervous system.

Develop an Ability to Say 'No' Visualise yourself saying no to comfort foods.

Distract yourself Develop a list of non-food-related activities (short activities that take no longer than 10-20 mins to complete) that you can do to take your mind off the craving e.g. take a warm bath, walk around the block, paint your nails, check your emails, read a book etc.

These practical strategies for overcoming food cravings tend to work best if practised regularly. Keep in mind that everyone at some point has food cravings and so. to a certain extent, they are a normal part of our everyday hectic lives. Cravings can, however, come under some level of personal redirection so that we do not have to succumb to them every time and therefore jeopardise our health.

Take Home Points

Cravings are caused by our appetite.

- Our appetite can result from a desire to appease a negative emotion or stress, from a positive food association with a certain memory, or from habit.
- To overcome our cravings we need to balance our brain chemistry including identifying any deficiency in 3 common brain neurochemicals - noradrenaline, serotonin and dopamine. These can become deficient due to stress, fatigue, depression, anxiety, chronic illness, as well as individual personality and genetic factors.
- We can also try some simple practical strategies to overcome cravings, including removing temptation, avoiding being too hungry, being prepared, identifying our trigger times, and by practising the 'Five Ds'.
- Food cravings can be considered to some degree a normal part of our lives, especially as food is so much in abundance these days.
- Cravings do not, however, have to rule your life or ruin your health. As long as these cravings are tempered with mostly healthy eating and kept to a minimum you will find that succumbing to a food craving occasionally will not get you too far off track with your health goals.

YOUR *Weekly* CHALLENGE . . . .

This week your challenge is to learn to overcome your food cravings by either balancing your brain chemistry and/or by applying some of the practical strategies suggested in this chapter.

say die to dieting forever

This might seem a harsh statement but dieting really does more harm than good. It can be hard to accept this when we are desperate to achieve weight loss. Often we feel that we need to diet to stay motivated, to kick-start our healthy eating plan or to start seeing results. The reality is, however, that with only 5 per cent of individuals being able to maintain the lost weight from dieting it appears that diets do not work in the long term[1]. In fact, most individuals regain the weight plus extra kilos following dieting due to a change in their appetite, metabolism and body fat levels. So how does dieting fail?

Health FACT ·····································

You have not failed when you are unable to continue with a diet, the diet has simply failed you.

Why Dieting Will Always Fail You

The key to achieving a healthy weight for your frame is to never diet. We are biologically programmed to not diet as this is seen as a major threat by our bodies to our own survival. After all, from our bodyies' perspective, famine is something to be feared at all costs. Dieting essentially tells your body that it is currently experiencing a terrible period of famine. As a result, internal body mechanisms are put into motion to prevent the weight from easily coming off in the first place and then to quickly cause us to regain the weight once we have stopped dieting.

In fact, studies reveal that during dieting our hunger centre is activated so that we have insatiable appetites and our body turns a blind eye to how much body fat it feels comfortable carrying. Normally the amount of body fat we are carrying is tightly regulated and our hunger is kept under control through hormones called 'leptin' and 'ghrelin'. These hormones keep our body fat stores in check as a way of safeguarding our survival. When we have periods of dieting these hormones can get thrown out of balance and send signals to our body to increase our body fat stores to protect us from the next 'famine'. This means that when you have returned to normal eating you will gain even more weight than when you started.

The Yo-Yo Dieting Mindset

This brings me to another major reason diets do not work in that we are forced to eat a certain way that is not 'normal' for us. When we start a new diet we may be deprived of our favourite foods or the diet may be unrealistic to maintain and not flexible. For example, not wanting to be excluded from enjoying social events we succumb to eating our favourite foods and then feel like we have failed our diet. This can start a cycle of yo-yo dieting, which goes something like:

1 Decide to stick to a set diet plan
2 Succeed in doing this for a period of time
3 Start seeing results and getting compliments from others
4 Feel like a success
5 Start feeling deprived and/or hungry
6 Succumb to temptation and eat our favourite foods
7 Overeat or binge eat
8 Feel shame and guilt
9 Decide to stick to the diet again tomorrow or on Monday
10 Fail again at sticking to the diet soon after
11 Feel like a failure

This can be a dangerous cycle and lead to ever-increasing weight gain and low self-esteem.

Further to the psychological pulls of dieting there are real physiological disruptions caused by dieting that essentially put into motion metabolic and biological blockades to stop you losing weight and to make you gain it back again. In essence, dieting activates 'thrifty genes' that induce weight gain, both by increasing your hunger drive and decreasing your metabolism, and dieting triggers other weight-gain mechanisms, many of which will be beyond your conscious control.

The fundamental drive behind these occurrences is that your body sees weight loss as a threat to survival; after all, having body fat protects you from dying from starvation, it cushions your organs, and keeps you fertile. In essence, having body fat is a sign of having enough to eat and thus being in an advantageous situation. Of course we know that being well-fed does not mean well-nourished. As discussed in other chapters, food has changed so much in recent times due to processing that many of the nutrients that signal satiety have been stripped from our foods. This means that we can be eating enough basic Calories but nourishment from our food is lacking; essentially our body will continue to crave more and more food, and weight, then, continues to rise.

Aside from balancing your food intake to include foods that contain nourishment, it is important that we learn how to eat in a way that is not depriving or condemning our bodies. Thus, a better approach is to not diet but develop a low-sacrifice healthy way of eating (explained further below). This will lead to positive changes in the long-term to our waistlines and confidence levels.

A Closer Look at Fad Diets

There are many fad diets out there that report amazing results, but these are usually fraught with misleading claims. There is no one type of diet that suits everyone. In fact, the best diet is the one you do not know you are on. Find an eating plan that works for you and that is both sustainable and enjoyable. For a list of common fad-diets currently promoted see Appendix B.

> *Health* TIP . . . .
> The best diet is the one you do not know you are on.

The Better Approach is Low-Sacrifice Eating

In his book *Weight Loss for Food Lovers*[2], Dr George Blair-West explains that there is a better approach to eating that helps to break the dieting mindset called 'low-sacrifice eating'. In this approach he states that the first step is to recognise foods that you cannot do without. This might be chocolate or coffee, for example. These are coined your 'high-sacrifice foods' because to give them up would involve a high level of personal sacrifice. His suggestion is to not remove these entirely from your diet but to make sure you include a small amount regularly as a way to curb cravings and therefore curb binge eating. The best time to eat these, according to Dr Blair-West, is for morning tea. That way you are less likely to overeat these foods and will crave them less in the afternoon or evening as you have already had your 'fix' for the day.

Admittedly, initially you may overeat your favourite food as you are so used to feeling guilty about eating it that when you give yourself permission to eat unrestrained you may overindulge. This is a normal psychological response to loosening the reins on controlled eating and is a sign that you have been restricting your food intake too much. If you find yourself initially bingeing on your high-sacrifice foods, make sure you do not then devote yourself to not eating them ever again. This only creates a cycle of deprivation and binge eating. Allow yourself to have a small amount again tomorrow or the next day – that way you break this cycle.

Removing Moral Labels From Your Food

Food does not hold any moral value yet when we attribute the labels 'good' and bad' to foods we inherently feel positive or negative about ourselves when we eat those foods. This can create a vicious cycle of feeling ashamed of our behaviours and who we are based on our food choices. This can set us up to binge eat and eat in secret, all of which can entrench in us an inability to have a healthy relationship with food. Other terms such as calling foods 'junk', 'naughty' or 'treats' can also attach connotations that are not helpful when it comes to establishing a healthy relationship with food.

More helpful and positive terms would be to label foods as 'sometimes' and 'everyday'. This means that all foods are permissible but not all foods may be beneficial to have every day. Thinking of foods in this way takes away the guilt factor and allows us to enjoy our food.

If Not Dieting Then What Do You Do?

As we learn to live in balance with our hunger cues, our appetites, and our bodies, we find that we will naturally gravitate towards foods that make us feel good. Often these are foods that are fresh and unprocessed. When our hunger regulation mechanisms are working efficiently we will eat until we are full and satisfied and then not think about food until the next meal. In essence we have moved towards eating based on our intuition and not based on a particular diet.

The healthier approach to weight management, then, is to not diet but to realise that our body wants us to be healthy and to be comfortable. If we shift our thinking away from needing to behave in an overly disciplined and controlled fashion in order to enjoy good health then we will automatically start to move towards this over a period of time. Depending on how long you have been out of sync with your body and hunger cues will determine to some extent how long your body will take to recalibrate. But it will do so, eventually, if you remain steadfast and refuse to diet and choose to live by the sound health principles laid out in this book.

Is Bariatric Surgery Really Your Best Option?

Just a word about bariatric surgery, which is an increasingly popular option for rapid weight loss. Although it can reduce weight it does not come without risks or complications. It also does not change your appetite for the foods you used to enjoy but will restrict your ability to eat these. The result is feeling frustrated and potentially depressed. It is not unusual for patients to explain to me that they would give anything to be able to eat a steak again or enjoy their favourite meal without feeling nauseated or experiencing abdominal pains. Consider seriously whether this is your only option if you are at a crossroads with your weight. Perhaps hold off and implement the principles in this book first and see if your weight is still an issue for you.

Take Home Points

Dieting just does not work in the long-term.

- Many individuals have attempted to diet but found they regain the weight they lost soon after returning to their usual eating patterns.
- The problem with dieting is that it sets in motion a cascade of biological factors that cause our hunger to go up, our metabolism to go down, and our body to do whatever it needs to regain that weight.
- A better approach is to practise a low-sacrifice way of eating, which means that you do not give up your favourite or 'high-sacrifice' foods.
- You can still incorporate your favourite foods into your diet without compromising your health or weight.
- Avoid morally labelling foods as 'good' or 'bad' as this can attribute unnecessary guilt when you eat foods that are labelled 'bad'. A healthier approach is to consider foods as 'everyday' and 'sometimes' foods.
- Bariatric surgery does not come without risks and these need to be considered seriously before going under the knife.

YOUR *Weekly* CHALLENGE . . . .

This week your challenge is to say 'die' to dieting forever. Try practising guilt-free low-sacrifice eating as explained in this chapter. Tune into your hunger cues and really learn to satisfy your body's needs by developing your sense of intuition when it comes to eating and food.

be healthy at any size

You can be healthy at any size! Current research suggests that in order to be healthy you do not have to be a certain size[1]. In fact there are plenty of individuals who are above their most comfortable weight who are very healthy; just as there are individuals who are thin but very unhealthy. By concentrating on wanting to be a particular size a shift can occur where instead of focussing on being as healthy as you reasonably can be you become trapped in food preoccupation, self-hatred, eating disorders and yo-yo dieting. These in the long run will be much worse for your emotional and physical health than carrying a few extra kilos.

Health TIP

Our body naturally wants to return us to a healthy weight for our frame. We should try to give it the right physical and mental conditions to do so.

Keep in mind, too, that before the early 1940s there was no standardised sizing. So wanting to be a size 10 or 12, for example, was a foreign concept because, at that time, clothes were made or altered by a tailor to fit you. The standardisation of clothing sizes only occurred with the industrialisation of the clothing industry and the need to make large amounts of factory-standard clothing. This meant that specific sizing of clothes needed to be developed. Unfortunately, society has personalised this and made it an enviable goal to be able to fit into smaller-sized clothing. But what this overlooks is that everyone's body shape is different and fitting into smaller sizes does not mean that you will necessarily be healthier.

Health at Every Size

Consider that your body will naturally want to be healthy at your given weight, regardless of what your current size might be[1]. Losing weight is not necessarily the answer, with research suggesting that being healthy is more about your health behaviours than it is about the number on the scales. This means that although your weight and size might not shift, by being intentional about improving your overall health and well-being through positive habits and lifestyle changes your body responds by working better. Of course, loss in body size might well be a natural effect of healthier behaviours but it should not be the focus.

Recognising that you can be healthy at any size does not serve as a reason to continue to live with unhealthy habits - quite the opposite. By focussing on your health behaviours as opposed to your weight and size you can be in tune with when you need to change your habits to feel healthier rather than just to look a certain way. This means that even if you are within what is considered a 'normal' weight range for your height you may still be quite unhealthy due to your behaviours not fostering a true internal health.

Consider evaluating your health by different measures. Healthy for you might mean, for example, having enough energy to do what you like doing and to feel good. It might also mean living without chronic diseases and having sound mental health. Whatever the focus might be for you try to steer away from a weight or size goal as this does not equate to good health, greater intimacy or happiness in the long run.

Why BMI Is Flawed

BMI (Body Mass Index) is a clinical measure of our body mass relative to our height. Unfortunately, many a time, individuals are quickly labelled 'overweight' or 'obese' based on this categorisation system and its tight BMI cut-off values. Similarly, those individuals who are below a certain 'healthy' cut-off BMI are considered 'underweight' or 'very underweight'.

One problem with BMI is that it does not take into consideration muscle mass, bone density, frame, gender or ethnicity. There are individuals, for example, who have plenty of muscle tissue and very little body fat who meet the criteria for obese on the BMI scale. The typical example of this would be bodybuilders and those who work out at the gym regularly.

The other problem with BMI is that it does not directly equate to health. Having a high BMI does not automatically make you less healthy than someone with a lower BMI. The best person to judge your health, in my opinion, is you. Rather than relying on an arbitrary value to determine whether you are of a healthy weight consider whether you

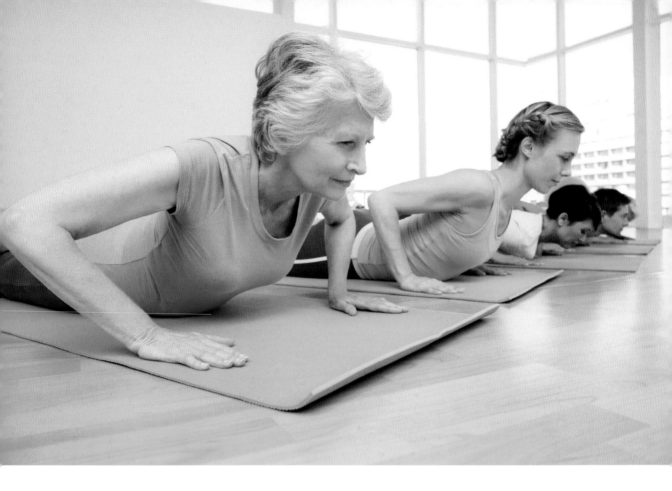

feel that you are living consistently with good health. If you are, then instead of relying on a particular weight or BMI-value determine to continue to evaluate your health based on how you feel.

Of course, it is still a good idea to get an annual or at least two-yearly health check for those asymptomatic health conditions that can affect any one of us and that we may not be aware of (as explained in Simple Health Habit #31 Have a Health Check).

Living Healthy Whatever Your Size

The first step in moving towards health is to accept that your weight may not change. In fact you might already be sitting at a healthy weight for your age and frame. Saying that, if you provide your body with what it needs, and let it do its job, which is to heal, sustain your life, and provide you with energy, it will naturally return you to a healthy weight.

The Health at Every Size movement[1] supports this notion and began in full swing in the late 60s. It is based on the premise that the best way to improve your health is to honour your body. It supports people in adopting health habits for the sake of health and well-being (rather than weight control).

Health at Every Size therefore encourages:

- Accepting and respecting the natural diversity of different body sizes and shapes.
- Eating in a flexible manner that values pleasure and honours internal cues of hunger, satiety and appetite.
- Finding the joy in moving your body and becoming more physically vital.

In essence, the premise of being healthy, no matter what your size, is to take the focus off weight and focus instead on good health and feeling great.

Take Home Points

Research suggests you can be healthy at any size.

- This means that you can enjoy your body for what it has to offer and enjoy good health regardless of what the scales tell you.
- Many individuals cease living a happy life because they are waiting to be a certain size.
- The reality is if we take the focus off weight and focus instead on living out the healthiest expression of ourselves then our body will return to a comfortable weight; all the while enjoying our lives to the full.
- Although BMI can provide a guide to how our weight is in relation to our height, it is often inaccurate.
- A better approach is to gauge your health based on how you feel.
- The Health at Every Size movement supports body acceptance for everyone and the view that health habits can be adopted for the sake of health and well-being rather than for weight control.

YOUR *Weekly* CHALLENGE . . . .

This week your challenge is to practise gauging your current health on how you feel and asking yourself whether your lifestyle is consistent with the healthiest expression of you that is possible. Take the focus off your weight and place it on feeling healthy and well.

stay regular

Keeping our digestion moving is so important. Many people have problems in this area. In fact, problems with a sluggish bowel and constipation affect around 2-10 per cent of the general population and up to 23 per cent of older adults[1]. It is a more common problem in women than men[1]. Not only can being irregular cause abdominal discomfort but it also comes with other significant health problems.

What are the Symptoms of a Sluggish Bowel?

- Not passing a bowel motion at least every second day (ideally daily)
- Hard stools that are difficult to pass
- Stools that are pellet-like (see Bristol stool chart[2] - ideal stools are Type 3 or Type 4)
- Pain with passing a bowel motion
- Pain after passing a bowel motion

Bristol Stool Chart

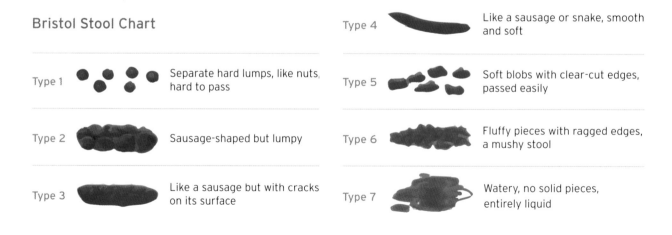

| Type 4 | Like a sausage or snake, smooth and soft |

| Type 1 | Separate hard lumps, like nuts, hard to pass |

| Type 5 | Soft blobs with clear-cut edges, passed easily |

| Type 2 | Sausage-shaped but lumpy |

| Type 6 | Fluffy pieces with ragged edges, a mushy stool |

| Type 3 | Like a sausage but with cracks on its surface |

| Type 7 | Watery, no solid pieces, entirely liquid |

- Bright red blood in your stool
- A history of haemorrhoids or anal fissure (tearing)
- Abdominal discomfort or pain
- Fatigue and generally feeling unwell

Long-Term Health Issues of Having a Sluggish Bowel

The issue with having a sluggish bowel long-term is that it can lead to the following health concerns:

Diverticular disease Is a common condition that results in stretching of the large bowel wall leading to the development of pouches in the wall. These pouches collect faecal matter and can become infected. This infection is called 'diverticulitis'. Around 5 per cent of 40 year olds have diverticular disease and this number increased to around 30 per cent of 60 year olds[3].

Faecal incontinence Loss of the ability to control bowel motions. This can be a significant problem and affects around 1 in 20 people[4]. Constipation can be a significant contributor and/or exacerbating factor in the development of faecal incontinence.

Pelvic floor weakness Straining to pass bowel motions, which can weaken the pelvic floor. This can lead to pelvic discomfort and problems with rectal prolapse.

Haemorrhoids Straining can cause weakening of the rectal veins in the anal region. When this happens, small grape-like structures called haemorrhoids form internally and/or externally in the anus/rectum. These can be itchy, painful, and bleed when passing a bowel motion.

Anal tearing (fissure) Straining can cause tearing of the anus. This causes pain and discomfort when passing a bowel motion.

Bowel cancer Long-term constipation has been linked to bowel cancer and tumours of the bowel[5].

Bowel obstruction When the bowel becomes blocked with hard faecal matter it can become obstructed to normal flow. This causes severe pain and in some cases can lead to death from bowel perforation.

What Causes a Sluggish Bowel?

A sluggish bowel causes constipation. Constipation usually happens because the colon (part of the digestive system) absorbs too much water from your food. If the food moves through the digestive system too slowly, too much water may be absorbed. The bowel motions at the end of the digestive process are then too dry and hard.

Many things can cause or worsen constipation including:

- Not eating enough fibre
- Not drinking enough water
- Not doing enough exercise
- Anxiety, depression and/or grief
- Underactive thyroid
- Delaying the urge to go to the toilet
- Using laxatives for more than a few days at a time
- The side-effects of some medicines (even some common medicines like painkillers or iron tablets)
- Pregnancy
- Being overweight
- Some nerve diseases
- Some bowel problems like irritable bowel syndrome (IBS)
- A slow-transit bowel, which means it takes longer for the faeces to travel all the way to the rectum, so more water is removed over time and constipation is much more likely. This occurs where there is nerve damage such as with stroke, Parkinson's, multiple sclerosis or trauma.

How You Can Prevent a Sluggish Bowel

The best approaches to prevent a sluggish bowel, and therefore constipation, are the following simple strategies:

- Drinking 6-8 glasses of water per day helps to move contents in the bowel along and prevent constipation.
- Increasing fibre intake to 25-35 grams per day by having 2 serves of fruit, 5 serves of vegetables, some legumes and pulses, and plenty of wholegrains. Note that the more processed foods are the less fibre they contain). Increase fibre in your diet slowly to avoid bloating and excessive passing of wind. Always increase water intake when you increase fibre to avoid initial worsening of constipation.
- You may have heard that there are two types of fibre – soluble and insoluble. Soluble fibre is one that dissolves in water and helps with lowering cholesterol levels. Soluble fibre is found in fruits and some vegetables. Insoluble fibre acts as roughage for the bowel to keep things moving. This type of fibre is found in the skins of fruits and vegetables, as well as in wholegrains. Both types of fibre are important for different reasons. Making sure your diet is rich in the above foods will ensure you are getting enough of each type of fibre.

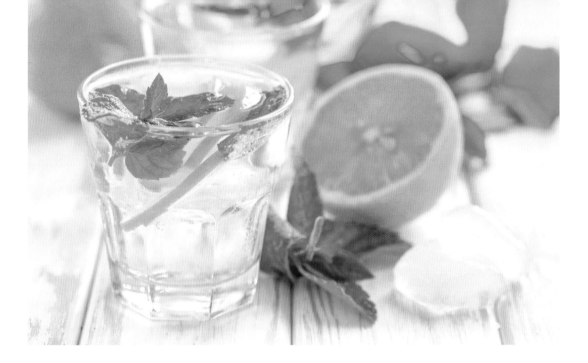

- Try to do some form of exercise on most days. This will help stimulate bowel movement. Walking for 30 minutes a day is an excellent way to meet this requirement.
- You can train your bowel to signal an urge to pass a bowel motion at a fairly regular time of the day by making sure that you never ignore the urge to pass a bowel motion as well as allowing sufficient relaxed time following the morning or evening meal to pass a bowel motion. Adopting the correct position to pass a bowel motion will help with avoiding straining. This involves sitting on the toilet with torso slightly leaning forward but back still straight, abdomen relaxed forward, and making sure your hips are flexed to a 90 degree angle to your thighs (sometimes using a small stool under your feet helps to achieve this).

Health TIP

Fruits high in fibre are usually those with an edible skin such as pears, apples, stone fruit and kiwi fruit.

Should You Take Laxatives?

Laxatives are commonly used in the treatment of constipation when the above lifestyle measures have not worked. The issue with taking laxatives is that they can make the bowel 'lazy', which can mean you become dependent on laxatives to pass a bowel motion.

You will find that your bowel will need more and more laxatives in this case to achieve the same effect as time goes on. There are a number of laxatives available on the market, but the safest are the bulking agents based on fibre such as psyllium husks, Metamucil, and Benefibre. Adding 1-2 tbps a day to your breakfast might be a helpful strategy if constipation is still an issue for you.

Magnesium oxide can also be a helpful agent in the treatment of constipation. Be careful not to take too much as it can cause abdominal cramping. The usual dose is 500-2000 mg a day. If these strategies fail to take effect see your health practitioner to ensure you are receiving the correct treatment rather than purchasing further over-the-counter laxatives.

Take Home Points

A sluggish bowel and constipation is a very common problem.

- Symptoms of a sluggish bowel include straining to pass a bowel motion, infrequent motions, pebble like motions, abdominal pains, blood in stool, and anal pain.
- Long-term constipation can cause other health concerns such as diverticular disease, faecal incontinence, pelvic floor weakness, haemorrhoids, anal tearing, bowel cancer, and bowel obstruction.
- There are many causes of a sluggish bowel but the most common include not drinking enough water, not eating enough fibre, and not doing enough exercise.
- To help prevent sluggish bowels the best strategies include drinking 6-8 glasses of water per day, increasing fibre intake to 25-35 grams per day, adopting correct bowel habits and doing some regular physical exercise,.
- If needed, laxatives can be used short-term to help restore normal bowel function. The safest are the bulking agents containing fibre such as Metamucil.

YOUR *Weekly* CHALLENGE . . . .

Your challenge this week is to stay regular. Try to increase water intake to at least 6-8 glasses per day, increase your fibre intake to 25-35g per day, and undertake some regular physical activity on most days of this week. If you need to, add 1-2 tablespoons of psyllium husks or Metamucil to your breakfast to increase fibre intake and bulking of your stools.

digest well

Poor digestion is a major contributor to not feeling well. The important thing to realise about digestion is that what goes in should not resemble what comes out! Food should be completely broken down in the gut and most of the nutrients should be absorbed. Indigestible waste products should be the only things that are the end product of a functional digestive system. When our digestive system is not working well, however, the end result is a range of symptoms that can be debilitating. The key to fixing our digestive system lies in understanding how it works and diagnosing any underlying issues.

Health TIP

When it comes to digestion what goes in should not resemble what comes out! Food should be completely broken down by a healthy digestive system.

Signs & Symptoms of Poor Digestion

The following signs and symptoms can indicate that our digestive system is sick and in need of attention:

- Heartburn
- Reflux
- Fatigue
- Bloating
- Abdominal pains
- Loose or hard stools (refer to Bristol stool chart in the previous chapter)

- Mucus in your stools
- Excessive wind
- Undigested food seen in your stools
- Feeling of incomplete emptying of bowel

If any of the above only occur for a short period of time then there is no real concern. But when we have ongoing signs and symptoms of digestive health issues then we have a problem. To understand what exactly causes these digestive issues it is important to understand in simple terms how the digestive system functions.

How Healthy Digestion Works

Digestion begins in the mouth. The first step in breaking down our food is to chew it properly. Chewing not only mechanically breaks down our food but also stimulates the release of certain enzymes that help to further digest starchy foods like bread, pasta and other carbohydrates.

The next step in the digestive process is swallowing effectively so that food is passed on to our stomach. The acidity in our stomachs allows proteins in our food to be broken down. Food in the stomach is pummelled and compressed until it is a dough-like consistency. It is then passed onto our small intestine.

In the small intestine, bicarbonate is released to neutralise the acid from our stomach. This allows pancreas enzymes to be activated in the small intestine, which further breaks down our food. Bile is also secreted into the small intestine from the liver. Bile helps us to absorb fats in our diet. Food is then broken down further into very small molecules by the enzymes produced on the surface of our small intestine. The surface of the small intestine should resemble a shagpile rug, which greatly increases the absorption surface area of the gut. Once most of the food nutrients have been absorbed, the remaining products of digestion move to the large intestine.

The large intestine is responsible for absorbing water from our food and is also home to an environment of good bacteria. These good bacteria are essential to healthy digestion and produce some essential vitamins such as vitamin K, which is needed for normal blood clotting. Interestingly they also help to produce a hormone called 'serotonin'. This hormone acts on the brain and gut nervous systems to assist in improving brain and gut function. Serotonin is known as our 'happy hormone' and is key to preventing depression, but it also acts in the gut to keep the gut 'happy'.

The last step in digestion is to effectively eliminate the waste products as faecal matter. This should be an effortless process and not a painful or prolonged process. The whole digestive journey takes several hours and never stops, even when we are sleeping. So where exactly can this process go wrong and what causes digestive health issues?

Causes of Poor Digestion

Digestive issues can arise from a variety of different conditions - some serious - but by far the most common issues causing poor digestion are:

Mechanical Issues This includes problems that arise because we do not chew each mouthful of food enough times. If we are not chewing properly and/or chewing quickly (often whilst talking) we will not break down our food properly. Ideally we should be chewing each mouthful 20-30 times. For most of us that is 4-5 times more than what we are currently doing. The other issue with chewing quickly or talking whilst chewing is that we end up swallowing a lot of air. This can build up in our stomach and cause belching and problems with wind.

   The other mechanical issues that commonly arise are reflux and heartburn. These issues often arise because we have too much back-pressure on the valve at the top of the stomach. This valve is responsible for holding the contents of the stomach down. When we have eaten a meal that is too large, if we have excessive wind in our stomach, or even if we are carrying too much weight around our middles then this puts pressure on that valve. The result is a spilling of the stomach contents up into the oesophagus and sometimes even into the mouth.

Absorption Issues One of the most common issues with not being able to break down food, protein foods in particular, is the fact that we drink with our meals. When this happens we dilute our stomach contents and in particular lower the acidity of our stomach, which actually needs to be kept fairly constant to be effective at breaking down our food.

Inflammation Issues Inflammation in our digestive system can occur when something we are eating is not agreeing with us, as when we have a food intolerance. Inflammation can cause pain but also reduces digestion of our food. When this happens, the food we eat does not get broken down properly and ends up passing to our large intestines partly undigested. The bacteria in our gut then ferments the undigested food, particularly the sugars in our food, and creates gas. The result is that we feel bloated and in pain.

   When our gut is inflamed we also feel fatigued, lethargic and just not comfortable. Inflammation of our guts can also be the result of diseases such as Inflammatory Bowel Disease (IBD) or other autoimmune-type diseases. These often cause more severe symptoms.

Microorganism Issues Interestingly, gut health also relies on the microorganisms that live in our gut. These 'bugs' create a microscopic ecosystem that is either a healthy one or a toxic one. Many individuals have an imbalance between good and not so good gut bugs. There have been numerous studies to indicate that having the wrong balance of bugs in our gut can result in digestive health issues[1]. Imbalances in our gut microorganisms can arise any time in our lives including as early as infancy. They might be the result of not being breastfed as a baby or inheriting not-so-good bugs from our mum during our birth, or from taking antibiotics frequently as children or as an adult. Other factors proposed to cause this imbalance include stress, drinking chlorinated water, exposure to agricultural chemicals, being on the oral contraceptive pill and/or having poor diets high in sugar and processed foods.

Pathological Issues The pathological issues include diverticular disease, bowel cancer and other bowel tumours. All of these can cause some issues with gut function.

How Can You Find Out What is Wrong?

Diagnosing gut issues can be tricky. Irritable bowel syndrome (IBS), for instance, is considered a diagnosis of exclusion whereby other more life-threatening conditions have been ruled out. There is, however, a process to undertake in getting to the bottom of your gut issues including:

- Blood tests will check for signs of inflammation, food allergies, and something called coeliac disease (gluten 'allergy').
- Scans can identify series issues. Scans include ultrasound scans, X-rays and CT scans. Your local doctor will know which one, if any, you may need.
- Bowel studies include having a colonoscopy and/or endoscopy where a camera is passed into the small intestine up via the anus or down via the mouth, respectively.
- Stool tests check for the presence of harmful bacteria and other organisms. Most specialised testing can also check for imbalances in gut microorganisms, which can provide valuable information on the potential source of gut inflammation and digestive issues.

All of the above testing needs to be carried out by a medical professional. Once testing has been carried out, then a treatment plan can be formulated for you.

How To Treat Your Digestive Issues

Depending on the cause of the digestive issues the specific treatment will vary but some basic principles for improving digestion include:

- Chew each mouthful well and chew slowly.
- Avoid drinking with your meals.
- Digestion can be aided by adding apple-cider vinegar to your meals as a dressing
- Reduce your portion sizes to avoid overfilling your stomach
- Trial digestive enzymes if you find you are still having difficulties digesting. These can be found at most good health food stores and are taken as a capsule with main meals.

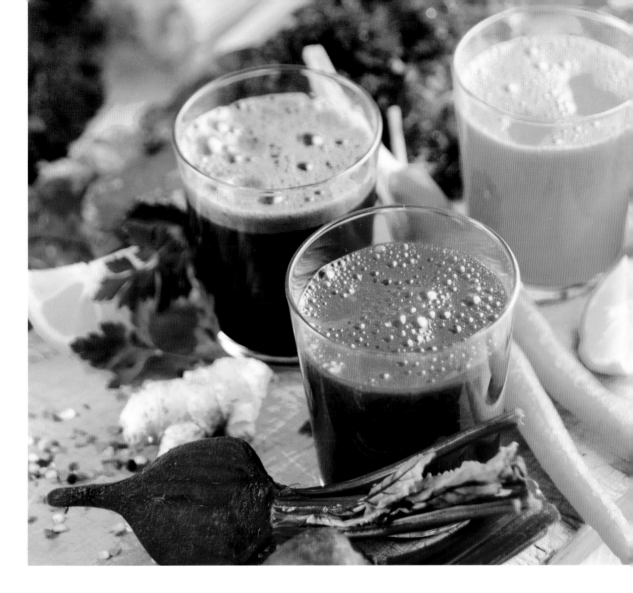

- Some individuals also find symptom relief by taking a product called Iberogast, which contains a number of herbs proven to help digestive symptoms such as heartburn, abdominal pains and cramping, and indigestion[2]. The usual dose for adults is 20 drops 3 times a day in ½ glass of water.

- There are many other products on the market that claim to assist in healing the gut. These include aloe vera products, glutamine and slippery elm. My general advice with these products is that anecdotally they do not seem to have any side effects so can be tried if other measures have not helped. Bone broths are said to also assist in healing the gut.

- Trial a good-quality probiotic for around 2–3 months. If you find that you have no improvement then consider trialling fermented foods instead of a standard store-bought probiotic. Fermented foods have been found to contain live cultures of probiotics in their most natural form[3]. Examples of fermented foods include sauerkraut, kefir, natto, kimchi, and other fermented products on the market (e.g. fermented papaya, fermented coconut water). Start by taking a very small amount of fermented foods and build up when you feel comfortable.

- If you are still struggling with debilitating gut symptoms there are medications on the market that may help including Mintec, Buscopan and Colofac.

Take Home Points

- Gut health is imperative to feeling well.
- Symptoms of poor gut health include bloating, abdominal pains, excessive wind, undigested food in your stools, diarrhoea or constipation and mucus in your stools.
- Digestion begins in the mouth and ends at the anus and involves a complex process of breaking down our food into smaller and smaller components so that microscopic food nutrients can eventually be absorbed into our bloodstream.
- There are many causes of gut health issues some of which are mechanical issues. Others involve functional and pathological components. IBS is a diagnosis of exclusion once other potential causes of gut dysfunction have been ruled out.
- Diagnosis of gut-health issues may involve having blood tests, scans, stool tests, and/ or a colonoscopy or endoscopy. Your medical health practitioner is the best person to guide this process.
- Treatment of gut-health issues depends on the underlying cause of the problem but ranges from simple measures like chewing slowly and not drinking with your meals, to more complicated treatment regimens that can be guided by a medical health practitioner.

YOUR *Weekly* CHALLENGE . . . .

Your challenge this week is to address your gut health. If you are having any issues in this area make sure you seek some professional medical advice this week. Even if you are not experiencing significant concern in the area of gut health, everyone can benefit from simple measures to optimise digestion, such as slowing down chewing and chewing food properly, not drinking with meals, and adding some apple cider vinegar to lunch and dinner as a dressing.

recognise food upsets

Many people nowadays suffer from either food allergies or intolerances. These general 'food upsets' can lead to some significant symptoms and can be debilitating for the sufferer. Food allergies and intolerances are on the rise, but medically the reason for this is yet to be determined. Many people with food upsets interestingly do not realise that they are indeed suffering from either an allergy or intolerance and just bear the discomfort. But effective management strategies exist to alleviate the symptoms of food upsets so it is worth exploring these.

Health TIP . . . .

Food Allergies = immune reaction to food proteins and can be life-threatening.

Food Intolerance = sensitivity to food chemicals and not life-threatening.

What Is A Food Allergy?

Food allergies happen due to an overreaction of the body's immune system to a food protein. Around 2 in every 100 Australian adults suffer from food allergies[1]. Most food allergies start in infancy or as a toddler and can be outgrown – such as egg and milk allergies, which are usually outgrown by the time children are school-aged. Food allergies do not appear to be genetic, but if you have a sibling with a food allergy then you have an increased chance of developing a food allergy also.

The symptoms of food allergy can be life threatening. The key feature, though, of an allergy is that the reaction occurs every time to even small amounts of the substance.

Common symptoms include:

- Iitching, burning and swelling around the mouth
- Runny nose
- Skin rash (eczema)
- Hives
- Diarrhoea, abdominal cramps
- Breathing difficulties, including wheezing and asthma
- Vomiting, nausea

The most common foods to cause an allergic reaction in a hypersensitive individual include (in order)[2]:

- Uncooked egg
- Peanuts
- Dairy
- Tree nuts
- Kiwifruit
- Sesame seeds
- Prawns and other crustaceans
- Wheat
- Fish

Food allergies are diagnosed by a skin prick test or allergy blood test. Sometimes these tests can come back 'false positive', which means that they have detected an allergy but you have never experienced any symptoms. In this case a food challenge may be required where you will be given small amounts of the food, under medical supervision, to see if you react.

What Is A Food Intolerance?

A food intolerance, on the other hand, is a 'chemical' reaction that some people have after eating or drinking certain foods; it is not an immune response. It essentially means that individuals are unable to properly digest that food, which can lead to bloating, pain and either diarrhoea or constipation. Surveys indicate that up to 25 per cent of the population believe they have some sort of food intolerance[2] and they often run in families, suggesting a genetic predisposition.

Food intolerance has been associated with asthma, chronic fatigue syndrome and IBS. It can cause significant symptoms which can come on hours or even days after you have eaten a particular type of food. This makes it difficult to pinpoint what exactly it is that you are intolerant to. Food intolerances can also get worse depending on how much of the food you have eaten.

People who have a food intolerance react to chemicals which either occur naturally in that food or are added to it during processing. Different people will tolerate different amounts of chemicals. The amount of the chemical that causes symptoms is called the 'dose threshold'. Some people have a high dose threshold to all food chemicals and may never have symptoms after eating foods. These people typically will never experience food intolerances throughout their life. Food intolerances can occur suddenly following an illness, change in diet, major life stress, pregnancy or surgical procedure.

More than one type of chemical may cause symptoms, so a person may react to many different types of foods. Some foods contain the same chemicals and a person can react after eating any of those foods. This is because the chemical slowly builds up in the body until the dose threshold is reached. It also explains why the same food does not cause symptoms every time it is eaten, because the amount eaten may not have been enough to cross the dose threshold.

Symptoms That Suggest You Have a Food Intolerance

Common symptoms of food intolerances include:

- Headache, migraine
- Abdominal pains
- Bloating with excessive wind
- Mouth ulcers
- Sweating
- Palpitations
- Diarrhoea
- Flu-like aches and pains
- Fatigue
- Mood changes
- Burning sensations on the skin
- Breathing problems – asthma-like symptoms

Food intolerances may be caused by sensitivity to the following natural food chemicals:

Salicylates These are naturally found in many fruits, vegetables, nuts, herbs, spices, jams, honey, yeast extracts, tea, coffee, juices, beer, wine, mint and fruit flavourings, as well as scents in perfumes, toiletries, cleaning products and washing powders. It is also found in aspirin. Also, the more unripe fruit is the more salicylates it contains.

Amines These are found in meats, fish and cheese especially as they age. So levels of amines will be higher in meat and fish that is not fresh as well as meat that has been slow-cooked or roasted. Amines are also found in ripe bananas, tomatoes, avocados, pawpaw and olives. High levels are found in tomato sauce, fruit juices, chocolate, nuts and seed pastes, and in fermented products such as yeast extracts, wine, beer.

Glutamates This is a natural amino acid found naturally in many foods and enhances the flavour of foods in cheese, tomato, mushrooms, stock cubes, soy sauce, meat extracts, and yeast extracts.

As well as to the following:

Lactose Milk sugar malabsorption is caused by a deficiency of the enzyme lactase. Levels of lactase are maintained for life in people of northern European background, but in those who are of Aboriginal, Asian, Mediterranean and Middle Eastern descent, levels fade during childhood. Drinking lactose-free milk may help to relieve symptoms.

Fructose Incomplete absorption of the sugar found in fruit, some vegetables (e.g. corn), honey, and table sugar. Having excessive amounts of fruit or concentrated fruit sugar such as that found in fruit juice and dried fruit can cause symptoms such as bloating, reflux, abdominal pains, wind and diarrhoea.

Short-chain Carbohydrates There can be a malabsorption of fermentable sugars contained in many different fruits, vegetables including garlic and onions, beans and pulses, wheat, rye, barley, sweeteners and chocolate. This is the basis of the low FODMAP diet as a management strategy for IBS as the majority of IBS sufferers are thought to have short-chain carbohydrate malabsorption with or without any other food chemical intolerances.

Gluten or Wheat Gluten intolerance is different to coeliac disease, which is explained below. An intolerance to gluten or wheat likely means you will experience bloating, abdominal pains, and wind when you eat large amounts of wheat. But in smaller amounts it may be tolerated. In coeliac disease no gluten or wheat is permissible.

Cow's Milk Protein Milk intolerance means intolerance to the A1 type of cow's milk protein but also sometimes the A2 cow's milk protein. This is usually seen in infants and children rather than adults. Drinking A2 milk may help with digestion.

Caffeine Acts as an irritant to the bowel.

Food chemical intolerances may also be to the following food additives:

• Preservatives

• Artificial food colours

• Flavour enhancers e.g. MSG

If you are sensitive to natural food chemicals you are usually also sensitive to at least one preservative, artificial colour and/or flavour enhancer. The ones that are likely to cause reactions are listed in Appendix C at the back of this book.

The diagnosis of food intolerance is more difficult than allergy as it will not show on a blood or skin-prick test. The best way to diagnose a food intolerance is by conducting an elimination diet. For more information on how to conduct a formal elimination diet refer to the Royal Prince Alfred Hospital Elimination Diet Handbook[3].

How to Manage Food Upsets

The easiest way to manage a food allergy or intolerance is to eliminate the offending food/s from the diet. Try keeping a symptom diary for up to 1 week. If there are particular foods that cause digestive upset, try avoiding them for at least 2 weeks to see if your symptoms improve. The most common food intolerances that I see in clinical practice are to gluten and dairy.

Health TIP ·

Look after your good gut bacteria by feeding them well. Sugars, food chemicals, and high levels of chlorine in water can all reduce the number of good gut bugs.

Following the low FODMAP diet for a period of time, in particular to reduce bloating symptoms, can be helpful[4]. Resources about the low FODMAP diet can be found on the Monash University Medicine, Nursing and Health Sciences website[4].

Although, food allergies and intolerances cannot be cured, the symptoms and severity of the reaction can reduce over time. Sometimes, the body can tolerate the food if it is avoided for a period then reintroduced in small doses, particularly for food intolerances. Before you eliminate or reintroduce foods, my suggestion would be to seek advice from a specialist dietician or nutritionist.

Desensitisation immunotherapy may be an option for food allergies as a way to reduce sensitivity to that food. This is performed by an allergy specialist.

It is important to note that the symptoms of food allergy and intolerance can also be caused by other conditions, so it is important to get a valid medical diagnosis.

Could You Have Coeliac Disease?

Coeliac disease is not an allergy, but does involve an immune-system response to foods containing gluten and tends to run in families. When gluten-containing cereals (like wheat, barley, oats, oat bran, rye) are eaten, inflammation of the gut occurs, resulting in poor absorption of nutrients. Major symptoms are mouth ulcers, gut upset, fatigue, anaemia, skin problems and/or weight loss. Some people have no symptoms at all.

Screening blood tests may be able to detect this condition but the definitive diagnosis requires an endoscopy and small bowel biopsy. Currently for coeliac disease, a life-long gluten-free diet is the only effective management strategy. Those who continue to eat gluten risk osteoporosis, chronic anaemia and/or bowel cancer.

Take Home Points

Food allergies and intolerances are common and appear to be on the rise for reasons not completely known.

- A food allergy occurs when the immune system reacts to a food protein. The most common food allergies are to eggs, peanuts, dairy, tree nut and seafood.
- Food intolerance occurs when the body has a chemical reaction to eating a particular food or drink.
- The symptoms of mild to moderate food allergy and intolerance may be similar, but food intolerances do not cause severe allergic reactions (such as anaphylaxis).
- The diagnosis of food allergies involves a skin allergy test or allergy blood test and the treatment is avoidance of the food. Sometimes immunotherapy desensitisation can be helpful in reducing food allergies.
- The diagnosis of food intolerances is more difficult and often involves a process of elimination of foods from the diet and then reintroducing them.
- Coeliac disease causes a reaction to gluten in grains such as wheat, oats, barley and rye. Complete life-long avoidance of gluten is the only current management strategy.
- It is important to recognise if you are suffering from a food upset as these can cause avoidable debilitating symptoms.

YOUR *Weekly* CHALLENGE . . . .

This week your challenge is to keep a food diary for several days and write down any symptoms such as bloating, fatigue, mouth ulcers, abdominal pain, diarrhoea, or constipation that you experience. If your symptoms are debilitating or you suspect that you might be suffering from a food upset consider speaking with your doctor about next steps in diagnosis.

love your liver & detox

Your liver is the key detoxification organ in your body and is situated on the upper right side of your abdomen, just below the ribs on that side. Along with removing toxins from the body, your liver processes food nutrients and helps to regulate body metabolism. This is why if your liver is damaged you start to accumulate harmful toxins in your body, you do not process food nutrients as efficiently, and your metabolism can really take a hit.

Health TIP . . . .

Our liver is the key detoxification organ in our body. If we want to feel well we must know how to look after our liver.

A range of conditions can prevent the liver from performing its vital functions. The one I see most in clinical practice is fatty liver disease and toxin damage. When our liver is not functioning optimally due to these situations we do not feel very well at all. In fact, it can so significantly impact our health that I have seen individuals completely debilitated by liver disease.

One patient in particular comes to mind. He was an otherwise fit gentleman of normal body weight but had found that, in recent years, he was overindulging in what he called 'the good life'. Too much alcohol, caffeine and café lunches had lead to some liver damage. His main symptoms were fatigue, itchy skin especially at night time, and an offensive taste in the mouth that he described as sometimes metallic. These symptoms were really starting to affect his quality of life to the point where he was taking time off work thinking he must be stressed. When he made some necessary lifestyle adjustments these symptoms largely resolved.

So what exactly are the functions of the liver and how do we restore and/or protect it so that it can continue to function well?

Functions of the Liver

The liver has over 500 essential functions to keep the body healthy. Some of those include[1]:

- Toxins, medications and drugs including alcohol are filtered through the liver and neutralised or converted into other forms by specific enzymes.
- Bile, produced by the liver, is stored in the gall bladder and used to help break down dietary fats. Bile is also needed in order to absorb the fat soluble vitamins A, D, E and K.
- The liver converts carbohydrates into glucose for instantly available energy and converts glucose into its storable form (glycogen). When blood sugar levels drop, glycogen is converted back into glucose.
- It synthesises cholesterol and produces the lipoproteins needed to transport cholesterol throughout the body, including low-density lipoprotein (LDL) cholesterol and high-density lipoprotein (HDL) cholesterol. Hence, when the liver is not functioning effectively, cholesterol levels begin to rise.
- The liver is the major fat-burning organ regulating fat metabolism. A healthy liver metabolises rapidly, keeping weight stable. A sluggish liver causes calories to be stored as fat rather than used for energy.
- Amino acids from protein are sent to the liver for the production of body proteins such as hormones.
- The liver changes ammonia (a toxic by-product of protein metabolism) into urea, which is then excreted in urine.
- It regulates blood clotting.
- It resists infections by producing immune factors and removing bacteria from the bloodstream.

Common Symptoms of Liver Damage

Symptoms of liver damage depend on the disorder, but can include[1]:

- Fatigue
- General malaise (feeling unwell)
- Nausea
- Vomiting

- Itching
- Diarrhoea
- Appetite loss
- Bloated abdomen, swollen ankles
- Abdominal pain in the upper right side
- Easy bruising
- Reduced immunity
- Jaundice (the skin or whites of the eyes turn yellow)
- Dark urine
- Fever
- Anaemia
- Changes in mental state – altered sleep pattern (awake at night), confusion, drowsiness.

How Can the Liver Be Damaged?

Some of the causes of liver damage include:

- Non-alcoholic fatty liver disease ('fatty liver') – results in fat accumulating inside liver cells, causing cell enlargement and sometimes cell damage. The liver becomes enlarged, causing discomfort on the upper right side of the abdomen. Fatty liver can occur if we are carrying too much weight for our frame, have diabetes, or consume too much sugar.
- Alcohol-related liver disease – alcohol is a toxin that, when consumed in excess, damages liver cells. In time this can lead to fatty liver, hepatitis and eventually cirrhosis of the liver.
- Toxic effect of medications, as well as some herbal medicines.
- Congenital or inherited abnormalities of the liver – involving accumulation of iron and copper in the body and some rare enzyme disorders.
- Hepatitis virus infections.
- Conditions leading to liver-cell and/or bile duct ('the plumbing system' of the liver) damage.

The most common cause of liver damage is fatty liver disease ('fatty liver')[1]. Cirrhosis is the end result of many liver conditions and involves severe scarring of the liver (with liver nodule formation). It is associated with a progressive decline in liver function resulting in liver failure.

How Can Liver Damage Can Be Diagnosed?

Liver disease is diagnosed using a number of tests, including:

- **Physical examination** The liver may be enlarged.

- **Medical history** Including medications and lifestyle factors such as diet and alcohol consumption, exposure to hepatitis viral infections, blood transfusions, tattoos or family history of liver disease.

- **Blood tests** To check the levels of liver enzymes and jaundice ('yellowness') and to assess the protein production capability of the liver. Along with an elevation in liver enzymes, other markers also elevate as a result of liver damage, including ferritin (iron stores), cholesterol and blood sugar levels. Sometimes blood tests do not reflect the fact that liver damage is in its early stages. If you have any of the above listed symptoms consider following the liver 'detox' advice below to see if you feel better.

- **Ultrasound scan of the liver** This will assess the liver size, check for any structural abnormalities and will detect fatty liver.

- **Other scans** Including computed tomography (CT) scan and magnetic resonance imaging (MRI).

- **Biopsy** A small piece of liver tissue is removed and examined under the microscope in a laboratory.

Once liver damage is detected, or even if liver damage is not picked up on blood testing but you have symptoms consistent with liver damage, the best way to restore optimal liver function is to provide an environment that will allow the liver to heal. This is often called a 'detox'.

How to Really Detox Your Liver

So how do you *really* detox your liver? There are many products available on the market that claim to help with detoxing the liver. There are also many diets that propose the same. The problem with many of these products and diets is that they are often expensive and not sustainable. As soon as you stop taking the product or following the diet and return to your usual lifestyle you will find the same problems occurring with your liver. To simplify the process of 'cleaning out' the liver I find the best strategy is to follow this 3-step process:

Remove Toxins The toxins that most often damage the liver are alcohol and common medications like paracetamol. Reduce the amount of these to within safe limits. The severity of liver damage will determine whether your physician will recommend you abstain from alcohol for a period of time to allow your liver to regenerate. Additionally, be cautious with the amount of caffeine you are consuming. In amounts up to 200 mg in adults (about 3-4 cups of coffee or tea) caffeine is a stimulant of liver function. Amounts of caffeine consumed above this, however, can also cause some liver damage.

Clean Up Your Diet Along with reducing alcohol, the other dietary change that you need to make to clear out your liver is to reduce the amount of processed foods and drinks you consume. Processed foods and drinks are often high in toxic fats such as trans fats and/or sugars, which are both equally damaging to the liver, but also contain preservatives, additives and artificial colourings. As these have no nutritional value at all but are seen as toxins, the liver has to work hard at eliminating them. Processed foods include items such as cakes, pastries, some cereals, biscuits, desserts, packaged fried foods and confectionary. Fresh is always best when it comes to the majority of foods we should be consuming. Processed drinks include soft drinks, energy drinks and flavoured milk drinks. Try and get used to drinking plain water.

Support Liver Function There are a few foods as well as natural medicine items that can help with supporting liver function. These include vegetables from the 'brassica' family - broccoli, kale, cauliflower, brussels sprouts and cabbage[2,3]. The protective effect of the brassicas is due to their high content of something called 'glucosinolates'. Once these vegetables are chewed and digested, glucosinolates are converted into two types of highly reactive compounds, which work together as powerful stimulants of the liver's detoxification pathways. Eating a serve of these types of vegetables regularly will help give your liver a boost. You can also purchase the brassica extract in tablet form. I feel, however, that nothing is a substitute for the real thing when it comes to food items, but this in an option for those who have significant liver damage and/or do not eat enough of these types of vegetables.

The other natural medicine item that is available with evidence indicating liver support is 'silymarin' (also known as 'St Mary's Thistle or milk thistle)[4]. This is an approved substance used in Europe for liver disease and can be taken even if you have mild liver disease. Always consult your physician, however, before taking any new substance, to ensure correct dosage and interaction with any other substances you may be taking.

Finally, as the liver and gut are intrinsically linked you cannot truly support liver function without supporting optimal gut function.

Take Home Points

The liver is the key detoxification organ in the body.

- When your liver is functioning well you will find that you will feel well, your energy reserves will be normal and your metabolism will be able to work efficiently (provided there are no other medical issues).
- Signs and symptoms of liver damage include fatigue, nausea, general feeling of malaise, itching, easy bruising, anaemia and pain or discomfort in the upper right side of the abdomen.
- The liver may be damaged due to toxin overload, poor lifestyle choices, some medications, some viruses, as well as due to some inherited conditions.
- Diagnosis of liver damage involves clinical examination, blood tests, ultrasound scans and sometimes a liver biopsy.
- The liver has amazing regenerative potential and can heal if provided a permissive environment in which to do so.
- To allow the liver to regenerate follow a healthy diet low in processed foods and drinks, with low to moderate caffeine and alcohol intake, and high in fresh vegetables such as those from the brassica family (broccoli, kale, cabbage, brussles sprouts and cauliflower).
- Silymarin is a herbal extract that may assist in supporting the liver and is available in various preparations.
- The liver must be supported with a healthy gut to function well

YOUR *Weekly* CHALLENGE . . . .

This week your aim is to love your liver! If you have not done so already, aim to reduce alcohol, caffeine and consumption of processed foods and drinks. Increase your intake of vegetables from the brassica family e.g. broccoli, cabbage, kale, brussels sprouts and cauliflower to at least 3 times this week (ideally 5 times).

say goodbye to toxic stress

Stress is toxic to our bodies. So toxic, in fact, that it poisons your body and mind to the point where you can be totally incapacitated. Worst of all, the effects of stress seem to creep up on you and leave you feeling worn out, depressed, anxious and overweight. In essence, stress can kill you softly. It has been estimated that 60-80 per cent of all the reasons that people see a GP are related to stress[1]. Such conditions include fatigue, headaches, inability to lose weight, mental-health issues, insomnia, digestive issues, muscle tension, difficulties conceiving, recurrent infections, and even high blood pressure, heart disease and cancer[2,3].

These health effects can take some time to recover from depending on how long you have been stressed and the type of stress you have been experiencing.

To illustrate how debilitating stress can be to your health I recall a patient of mine who came to see me due to unrelenting fatigue despite getting a good night's sleep. She was a busy working mum with 3 children. She ran her own business and tried to keep fit by running 3 times per week. Despite all the exercise she found she was unable to lose any weight but, in fact, was gaining weight steadily. She also found that her moods had changed - she was becoming more pessimistic and irritable. She often tossed and turned at night time and would wake up predictability in the night between 1-3 a.m. Despite eating fairly healthily most of the time her biggest weakness was caffeine and chocolate. She would drink on average 3-4 cups of coffee per day to stay awake and eat chocolate every night due to her sugar cravings. When she looked in the mirror she reported to me that she no longer recognised who she was. To add insult to injury people often told her she looked tired. So she came to see me in a desperate state of not knowing what was wrong. We discovered that her health was suffering under the effects of chronic stress.

Good Stress

It is important to realise that not all stress is bad. Some stress is actually good for you and helps to keep life interesting. Good stress is also called 'eu-stress'. We need just the right amount of stress to keep us motivated and challenged. Too little stress and we become apathetic and bored. But too much stress and that is where our health starts to suffer the consequences. The worse 2 types of stress are repeated stress and chronic stress. So what exactly are these and how do you avoid them from becoming toxic in your life?

Health TIP . . . .

To halt the stress response stop and take 10 slow, deep breaths. Repeat this several times a day and before sleep at night.

Repeated Stress & How You Can Reduce Its Effects

Repeated stress affects you on a frequent and recurrent basis. Common examples of things that can make you stressed include:

- Traffic
- Paying Bills
- Noise
- Crowds
- Sleep disturbance
- Isolation
- Loneliness
- Hunger
- Danger

This type of stress can be overcome by practising stress-reduction techniques such as taking 10 deep breaths, meditation, mindfulness, and regular, relaxing exercise such as yoga and/or Pilates. These types of activities activate our parasympathetic nervous system – which is literally our 'de-stress' nervous system. Practice makes perfect when it comes to winding down the stress response so try incorporating these stress-reducing activities daily.

But by far the worse type of stress is chronic stress.

Chronic Stress & How You Can Stop It Ruining Your Health

Chronic stress is a significant health-destroying component of our modern-day lifestyles. It literally drains your energy, speeds up ageing, lowers your mood and steals your health. So what is chronic stress?

When compared with repeated stress, which affects us on a regular basis but does ease off at some point, chronic stress is stress that does not seem to go away. It is the type of stress that happens, for example, when we are having relationship troubles, or not enjoying our job, or when we have a baby; when we are constantly worried about an issue in our lives, when we have suffered an injury or chronic illness, or even as a result of not sleeping well. The cause of chronic stress in our lives may be obvious or it may be subtle, but it has to be present consistently for at least 3-4 weeks to be classified as 'chronic'.

When this occurs our stress hormones start to rise. In particular, adrenalin and cortisol. Other hormones start to drop such as our sex hormones progesterone and testosterone, our happy hormone serotonin, and our metabolism-boosting thyroid hormones. There are some predictable and potentially debilitating symptoms that occur when there is this chronic change to our hormone levels as outlined in the table below.

HIGH ADRENALIN	HIGH CORTISOL	LOW PROGESTERONE (WOMEN)	LOW TESTOSTERONE (WOMEN & MEN)	LOW THYROID HORMONES	LOW SEROTONIN
Increased Blood Pressure	Increased Blood Sugar	Menstrual Period Problems	Reduced Sex Drive	Slowed Metabolism	Depression
Racing Heart Beat	Increased Cholesterol	Infertility	Reduced Muscle Repair	Tiredness	Anxiety
Breathlessness	Increased Tummy Fat	Mood Swings		Hair Loss	Insomnia (particularly waking between 1-3 a.m.)
Anxiety	Sugar & Salt Cravings	PMS		Dry Skin	
Panic Attacks	Fluid Retention	Impaired memory		Dry Hair	
Stomach Pains	Reduced Immunity	Worsened symptoms of polycystic ovaries, fibroids and endometriosis			
Nausea					
Excessive Sweating					
Dry Mouth					

Health FACT ·

If you are constantly feeling tired you may be suffering from a condition known as adrenal fatigue – this is a state of body burn-out.

So how do you stop chronic stress from ruining your health? The first thing to recognise is the major stress producers in your life. Make a list of these from 'most stressful' to 'least stressful'. Work on the top 2 most stressful first. Aim to see if there is anything about those situations that you can change, even if it involves counselling to change your perspective about the situation. Realise too that you can actually be addicted to stress. Learn to recognise when your life has gone from one drama to the next. Is there something in your life and personality that is attracting this type of chronic stress? This may be part of a deeper psychological condition that has roots in our upbringing or past and may need to be further addressed in the form of counselling.

Other techniques for reducing chronic stress include getting a good night's sleep, having regular 'time-outs' from your busy schedule, doing regular exercise, laughing daily, reducing caffeine and alcohol, forgiving others, developing positive relationships and meditating regularly.

When you have been stressed for a long period of time either constantly or repeatedly you can develop a condition known as adrenal fatigue.

How to Recognise Adrenal Fatigue

Ever felt absolutely exhausted for days, weeks, months or even years on end despite getting enough sleep? You may be suffering from adrenal fatigue. Adrenal fatigue occurs when we have been very stressed for a long period of time. When this happens we deplete our hormone levels to such as point that we are in a state of burn-out. Our adrenal glands are responsible for making stress hormones like cortisol, adrenalin and noradrenalin. These hormones are responsible for keeping us motivated, maximising our energy levels and allowing us to stay alert and active. What can happen over time, however, is that by constantly running on high stress levels we deplete these hormones.

So what are the symptoms of depleted stress hormones and therefore adrenal fatigue?

• Constant fatigue
• Feeling of weakness
• Dizziness
• Poor concentration
• Looking tired
• Irritability, depression and/or anxiety
• Stomach pains
• Joint and/or muscle pains
• Inability to lose weight and/or weight gain
• Sugar cravings

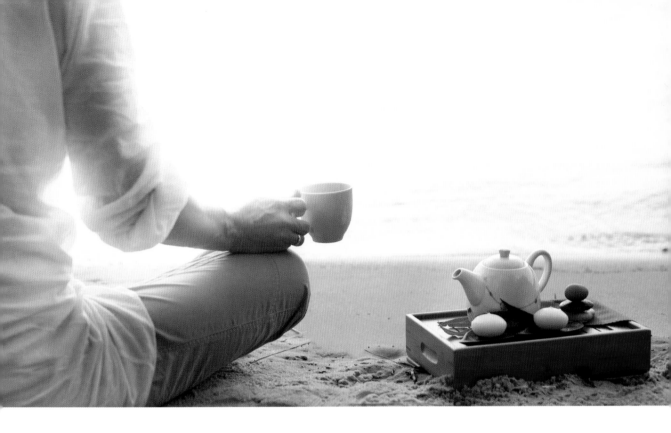

These symptoms can be subtle or can be severe and constant. So how do we reverse this process and return our stress hormone levels to normal?

- Realise that it will take time. It takes about 6–18 months to deplete our stress hormone levels and so it may take about this long to replenish them.
- Recognise our own limits when it comes to work and social activities.
- Make time to truly rest and recover.
- Clean up your diet by avoiding sugar, salt and fatty foods and eating mainly fresh, unprocessed foods.
- Eat small, regular meals every 2–3 hours to keep blood sugar levels stable.
- Reduce caffeine intake, which will only deplete stress hormones further.
- Avoid overtraining with exercise, which can worsen the situation. Learn to listen to your body when it comes to exercise. Gentle exercise such as yoga, Pilates and walking can be just as effective.
- Seek professional help when things aren't improving. Adrenal fatigue and the hormone imbalances that go along with this condition can be detected with some simple testing, including blood tests and salivary hormone testing. Depending on our symptoms and test results, our bodies may be in need of some additional support either with nutritional supplements or medications. Your medicine practitioner will be able to guide you in what you may need to help support your body.

So, to sum up, repeated and chronic stress is toxic to our bodies. Recognise when stress is ruining your body and mind and put measures in place to do something about it, even if this means seeking professional help.

Take Home Points

Stress that is long-term and repeated is toxic to our bodies.

- Symptoms of long-term stress include burn-out, fatigue, headaches, irritability, hormone issues, slowed metabolism, abdominal pains, muscle and body aches, sleep disturbances and recurrent infections.
- Some stress is a good thing and keeps us motivated and interested in our daily activities.
- Too much stress, however, can cause health issues including problems with fertility, reduced sex drive, weight gain, fluid retention, hormone imbalances, reduced mental concentration and anxiety and depression.
- If we have been stressed for a long time we can deplete our hormones to the point of burn-out. This state is particularly marked by constant fatigue, dizziness, sugar cravings and reduced mental concentration.
- The first step in healing our bodies from the effects of toxic stress is to recognise what our personal stress limits are and pull back from our work and other commitments if we are pushing ourselves too far.
- Put daily measures in place to reduce stress hormone levels such as taking 10 deep breaths, going for a walk, doing some meditation or yoga, praying, journaling, debriefing with a trusted friend, caring for a pet, or seeking professional help.
- Eating a healthy diet with reduced amounts of processed foods, sugar and caffeine will also help replenish energy reserves and avoid further symptoms of burn-out.
- Sometimes nutritional supplements and/or other medications are needed to help support our bodies if we have reached a state of 'adrenal fatigue'. These can be prescribed appropriately by a medicine practitioner.

YOUR *Weekly* CHALLENGE

This week your challenge is to put practical measures in place to reduce your stress levels. Whether this involves physically escaping from the stress (yoga, walking, a holiday, changing jobs or work hours) and/or mentally escaping from the stress (deep breathing, meditation, journaling, counselling, calling a friend, developing a hobby or caring for a pet). The key is to be consistent with these strategies this week.

avoid overstimulation

We certainly seem to be living in an overstimulated society and are constantly being bombarded by activities, forms of entertainment, social media and overflowing schedules. Not only are we in stimulation overload from external sources but we are also internally overstimulated as well. Many of the foods we eat, drinks we drink, and thoughts we think are overworking our bodies, minds, and, in essence, our souls. Every day I help individuals who say they feel tired yet wired – basically they are exhausted but cannot switch off their mind or body. Learning how to unwind and truly relax can be difficult, but it starts with avoiding overstimulation, which is essential to avoiding burn-out, anxiety and insomnia.

Health TIP . . . .

If you are feeling tired yet wired and find it difficult to relax or switch off at night consider you may be suffering from overstimulation.

What is Overstimulation?

Overstimulation involves exposing our minds and/or bodies to stimuli that is above and beyond what is healthy and appropriate for our level of tolerance. There are many things that can result in overstimulation but the causes I encounter most in clinical practice are:

- Internal Stimulants
  - Too much caffeine
  - Going to bed too late
  - Artificial colours, flavours and preservatives

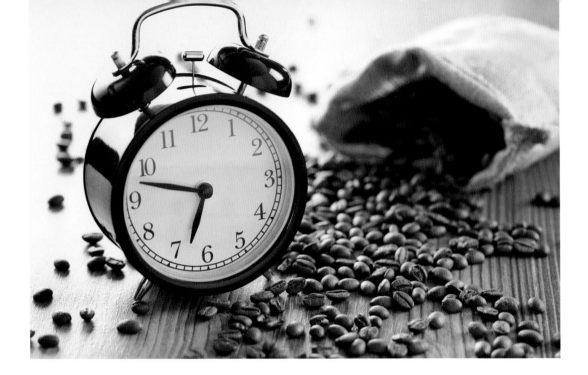

- Too much sugar
- Diet pills or supplements
- Excessive worrying
- External Stimulants
  - Social media
  - Television
  - Taking work home
  - No margin in your schedule
  - Work deadlines and pressures

In appropriate and evenly spaced amounts none of these things are harmful. In fact, our bodies are remarkably hardy and can tolerate quite a hit. The problem occurs when we have too many of these stimulants encroaching on our personal mental and/or physical space. Many individuals have so many of these things occurring on the same day that it has become their norm.

How Our Times Have Changed

Consider that 2 or so hundred years ago our lives were very different. We worked either in the home or on the land, usually in our family trade. We ate when we were hungry and rarely in excess due to limited supplies. Stress consisted of making sure there was enough food for your family and a roof over your heads. You slept when the sun went down and rarely stayed up past that hour as lamps and fires were expensive to run. Most of all, if people wanted to contact you they did so in person, wrote you a handwritten letter delivered on horseback, and they often stayed for a shared meal before the journey home. Our days did not consist of processed snacks, double-shot extra large skinny lattes, emails that seem to multiply with every click, meaningless social media updates, having to wear multiple roles and responsibilities, and having to share your time between work, home, television and endless social commitments. People had time to breathe, eat, sleep and live in peace.

How Do You Know If You Are Overstimulated?

If you ever feel the following consider that you may be suffering from overstimulation:

- Do you feel tired most of the time?
- Do you have difficulty switching off your brain at night?
- Do you feel exhausted but cannot sleep or rest?
- Do you feel agitated and unable to relax?
- Does worry and anxiety pervade your thoughts?
- Does your heart seem to skip beats or beat faster at times?
- Do you have headaches, a dry mouth, and/or muscle tension?
- Do you frequently fidget, cannot sit still, or feel uncomfortable with silence?
- Do you feel like you never have enough time?
- Do you feel energised after a meal or more tired?
- Do you use caffeine to give you an energy boost often?
- Do you feel like you want to give up but cannot due to responsibilities?

If you answered yes to any of these questions consider that you are likely suffering from overstimulation, whether it be from internal or external sources. Luckily this process can be turned around.

So How Do You Reduce Overstimulation?

The trick to reducing overstimulation is to firstly recognise what is really important in your life. Whenever a survey is undertaken asking individuals what their top 3 priorities in life are they usually list family as number 1, health as number 2, and financial security as number 3. Interestingly, we often neglect number 1 and 2 in pursuit of number 3. The irony is that too often I have seen this pursuit be in vain when the chase for success ends up costing people their health or their family. When I sense that people are really feeling the pinch of exhaustion and overstimulation I ask them to address what they value most in life. If they feel that it is spending time with family and feeling/being healthier I ask them to make some changes such as:

- Reducing the amount of time they watch television by ½.
- Reducing social media time by ½ or not engaging in social media until a set time in the day.
- Reducing the amount of caffeine they have in their diet by ½ and not having caffeine after 2-3 p.m..
- Avoiding dietary stimulants by reducing processed sugar by ½ in the foods they are eating and drinks they are drinking. By eating mostly fresh foods and drinking mostly water they meet this goal automatically.
- Going to bed before 10 p.m. each night, even if this means some work is left unfinished.
- Setting a reasonable 'to do' list at the start of the day with 6 items at most on that list.
- Learning to be assertive and say no to events and activities that are just not that important.
- Reducing the number of extracurricular activities by ½.
- Learning the art of truly relaxing. Taking some time to practise this each week. Sit in a comfortable chair, do some deep breathing, and focus on all the things in your life that you are grateful for.

I find that the above prescription really works to reduce the anxiety, stress and exhaustion that can come as an automatic by-product of living in today's frantic society.

Aside from the practical aspects of reducing overstimulation, if you are really finding it difficult to unwind and relax I have found that the following natural supplements can be helpful:

- **Magnesium** Taking a good-quality magnesium supplement before bed, either in tablet or powder form, can assist in relaxing the body. The best form of magnesium for absorption is citrate or biglycinate. Other individuals swear by topical magnesium in the form of Epsom salts in bath water at night to relax as well as in a lotion form to rub on after a shower or bath. Any of these forms of magnesium are worth a try.

- **GABA (short for gamma-aminobutyric acid)** This can be taken in tablet form and can greatly help individuals to relax. GABA is one of the chief relaxation neurotransmitters in the brain and works similarly to the benzodiazepine medications such as valium, but without the addiction potential. It should not be taken with valium.

- **Chamomile** This is commonly taken as a tea and many people swear by its effectiveness in helping them relax and sleep. It is safe to take, has no known side effects, and is even safe to take during pregnancy. Best of all, chamomile tea can be a great bedtime routine addition instead of another cup of black tea or coffee.

Take Home Points

We live in an overstimulated society where it is the norm to feel exhausted, overworked and overwhelmed.

- There are many stimuli which challenge our ability to maintain a manageable schedule, including social media, television, pressing deadlines and extracurricular activities.
- Along with external stimuli there are often internally derived stimuli that add insult to injury when it comes to being overstimulated. These include too much caffeine, too much sugar and processed foods, not getting enough sleep, as well as worrying about the future and about situations that we cannot change.
- Warning signs that you are suffering from overstimulation include feeling tired yet wired, not being able to relax or enjoy social occasions, feeling unfulfilled and frustrated, and not being able to prioritise your health or family.
- To unwind from overstimulation start by examining what your real priorities are. If they are different to what your current reality is then commit to making some changes to your schedule.
- Consider disciplining yourself to go to bed earlier, leave work at the office, reduce caffeine and processed foods, and switch off the television and social media at least 1 hour before bed.
- Some natural supplements that can help with relaxation and feeling overstimulated include magnesium, GABA and chamomile. Always speak to your health care practitioner first to ensure you are not causing problems by mixing medications or exacerbating any other health conditions.

YOUR *Weekly* CHALLENGE . . . .

This week your challenge is to reduce your level of overstimulation by $\frac{1}{2}$ by following the suggested strategies. Your mind, body and soul will thank you for making the change!

learn to breathe

Our body needs oxygen! This might seem like an obvious statement, but by observing how shallowly many of us breathe you would think we did not realise how much we need this vital element. Every cell in our body requires oxygen for a process called 'cellular respiration'. Of particular note are mitochondria, which are the powerhouses of our body as they produce energy from oxygen. When oxygen as a core ingredient is missing, the result is fatigue, muscle aches, and a range of other potentially debilitating symptoms. The key is to first learn how to deep breathe and then practise this often in order to well-oxygenate your tissues.

Health FACT . . . .

Did you know we breathe in and out around 300 times per day? That is around 8 million times in our lifetime.

What Is Deep Breathing?

Deep breathing involves moving air into the lower regions of your lungs instead of just the upper regions. This results in all regions of your lungs being well aerated and therefore able to absorb the maximal amount of oxygen.

The opposite of deep breathing is shallow breathing. When we shallow breathe the lowest portion of the lungs, which is where many small blood vessels instrumental in carrying oxygen to cells reside, do not receive enough oxygen. This can make you feel short of breath and even anxious. Not only can shallow breathing lead to reduced oxygen absorption into our bloodstream, it can also put us at risk of lower lung infections such as pneumonia.

How Do You Know If You Are Deep Breathing?

Deep breathing is also known as diaphragmatic breathing, abdominal breathing or belly breathing. That is, when you breathe deeply, the air coming in through your nose fully fills your lungs, and you will notice that your lower belly rises. This is because the act of deep breathing engages the diaphragm, a strong sheet of muscle that divides the chest from the abdomen. As you breathe in, the diaphragm drops downward, pulling your lungs with it and pressing against abdominal organs to make room for your lungs to expand as they fill with air. As you breathe out, the diaphragm presses back upward against your lungs, helping to expel carbon dioxide.

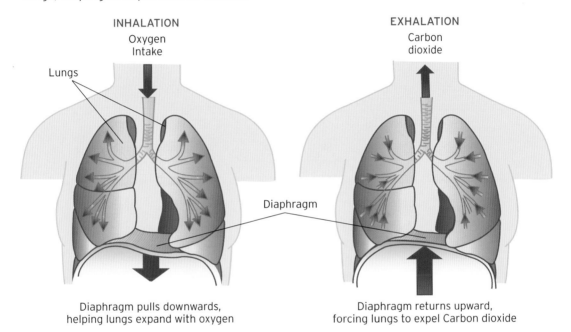

Image source: Harvard Health Publications[1]

    Shallow breathing reduces the diaphragm's range of motion. This means that our belly does not rise; instead our chest and shoulders rise.

    Deep abdominal breathing encourages full oxygen exchange; that is, the beneficial trade of incoming oxygen for outgoing carbon dioxide. Not surprisingly, this type of breathing slows the heartbeat and can lower or stabilise blood pressure.

Deep Breathing to Beat Anxiety

Our stress-and-anxiety nervous system, the sympathetic nervous system, is activated by shallow breathing. When we take small, shallow breaths our body thinks that we are in a state of alarm. The result is an elevation in heart rate, breathing rate and blood pressure. Along with this our brain starts to feel anxious.

Conversely, our 'de-stress' nervous system, the parasympathetic nervous system, is able to be activated by deep breathing. As a result our blood pressure, heart rate and breathing rate reduce. We feel calmer and less anxious. In essence, our sympathetic and parasympathetic nervous systems are acting in a tug-of-war. When one is active, the other is less active. If you are feeling tense, anxious or stressed start by taking 10 slow, deep breaths.

How to Deep Breathe Properly

Learning to deep breathe takes a little practice and self-observation. Firstly, find a comfortable, quiet place to sit or lie down. Start by observing your breath. First take a normal breath. Now try taking a slow, deep breath. The air coming in through your nose should move downward into your lower belly. Let your abdomen expand fully. Now breathe out through your mouth (or your nose, if that feels more natural). Alternate normal and deep breaths several times. Pay attention to how you feel when you inhale and exhale normally and when you breathe deeply. Shallow breathing often feels tense and constricted, while deep breathing produces relaxation.

Now practise deep breathing for several minutes. Put one hand on your abdomen, just below your belly button. Feel your hand rise about an inch each time you inhale and fall about an inch each time you exhale. Your chest will rise slightly, too, in concert with your abdomen. Remember to relax your belly so that each inhalation expands it fully. Count for 4 seconds as you breathe in, then pause as you hold the breath in for 2 seconds, and then breathe out for 3 seconds. Repeat this process 10 times for maximal effect. Do this every time you are feeling anxious, stressed, fatigued, or simply need to think a little more clearly. Your body will thank you for the extra oxygen by making you feel great!

Take Home Points

- Oxygen is a vital element required for every living cell in our body.
- When we deep breathe we oxygenate all areas of our lungs and allow for maximal absorption of oxygen into our bloodstream.
- When we are shallow breathing we can feel fatigued, tense, anxious, and even develop digestive issues.
- You can resolve anxiety by practising taking 10 slow, deep breaths whenever you are feeling uptight. This is because deep breathing activates our 'de-stress' or 'parasympathetic' nervous system.
- You know that you are deep breathing if your abdomen expands when you take a breath in.

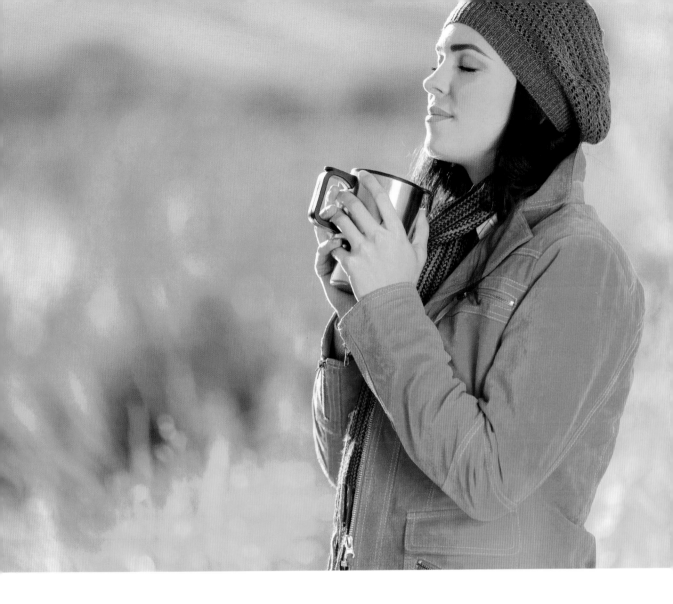

- Practise observing how you are breathing.
- Make a deliberate effort several times per day to deep breathe. Do this any time you are feeling anxious, tense, fatigued or worn out.

YOUR *Weekly* CHALLENGE . . . .

This week your challenge is to take time each day to take ten slow, deep breaths. Do this several times a day. For example, in the car on the way to work, before eating each main meal, and before going to sleep at night.

break negative thought patterns

We all think negative thoughts from time to time. However, if negative thinking becomes our habitual thought pattern then it can prevent us achieving true wellness and mental rest. Our thoughts are powerful determinants of our overall happiness and experience of life. When we dwell on negative thoughts for too long they can change our moods and emotions as well as our behaviours. In fact, we can even find that our negative thinking becomes a self-fulfilling prophecy. What we feared might happen can turn out to be the case just by way of natural gravitation towards that particular outcome. Saying that, negative experiences can happen without any input from us, but it is often our perspective that determines how that experience will ultimate affect us and our health.

Why Negative Thinking is Bad for Your Health

I meet so many patients who dwell on negative thoughts, whether it be about past experiences or potential future occurrences. They can become anxious and find it difficult to switch off their thinking at night when it comes time to sleep. The result is a downward spiral of fatigue and anxiety, which often results in them coming to see me for a sleep cure. Unfortunately, there is often no quick fix. The ultimate cure is about identifying and changing their thinking about a particular situation in their lives that they are worried about and are dwelling on.

Research has started to suggest that negative thinking can actually be toxic to our brain cells, causing inflammation and permanent damage[1]. This may lead to mental health conditions such as anxiety and depression as well as other brain conditions[1]. This suggestion that thoughts actually cause a release of toxic neurochemicals in our brains is a frightening one.

Sometimes negative thinking can be subconscious – you may not be aware that you are thinking a particular way. This is often due to the fact that thinking negatively has become a habit and a learned behaviour often passed down from our parents. It can be especially difficult to identify subconscious negative thinking. This is where some honest self-evaluation comes in.

It is important to identify if we have established conscious or subconscious patterns of negative thinking and to break these before they break our spirits and our well-being. Sometimes, especially if we have hit rock bottom, we need extra help in the form of cognitive behaviour therapy (CBT) delivered by a counsellor. As the name suggests this type of therapy looks to address how our negative thinking impacts our behaviours. So what are some common patterns of negative thinking?

Common Negative Thinking Patterns

NEGATIVE THINKING PATTERN		BREAKING THE HABIT
Mind reading	You think that you know what other people are thinking. Usually, you believe they think badly of you. You never check to see what they really think.	Try thinking the opposite. Assume everyone thinks well of you.
Fortune telling	You predict the way things will turn out in the future. Usually, you think things will go badly for you.	Try imagining a positive outcome. Assume everything will work out well.
Exaggerating	You exaggerate your mistakes and other people's successes. You think you are hopeless and will never be as good as anyone else.	Look at the facts. Everyone has good and bad qualities. Everyone makes mistakes sometimes and gets some things right. Remember that that includes you.
Tunnel vision	You focus on one bad thing and forget all the good things. You see one bad quality in yourself and ignore your good qualities.	Expand your view. Write a list of the good things. Spend some time thinking about them for a change.

table continues overpage

NEGATIVE THINKING PATTERN		BREAKING THE HABIT
Not counting the good	You reject good experiences by saying they do not matter. You use this as an excuse to hold onto a negative thought.	Accept the good things that happen in your life. Let go of negatives that weigh you down.
Labelling	You give yourself a negative label (I'm a loser) rather than just describing what went wrong (I made a mistake) or how you feel (I feel sad). You may do the same to others.	If you are feeling sad, say you are sad, but do not take the extra step of labelling.
Moving from emotion to fact	You assume your negative emotions are facts about the way things really are (I feel it, therefore it must be true).	Recognise that while emotions are real, they are internal and not facts about the world.
Should and must	You use 'should' and 'must' to push you along. You feel guilty when you do not meet them and angry when others don't.	Let go. Give yourself some breathing space. Accept that you cannot control the behaviour of others.
Personalising	You see yourself as the cause of some negative event, but you were not responsible for it.	Look at the facts. Let yourself off the hook.
Seeing it as all or nothing	You see things as all good or all bad. If you make a mistake, you see it as a total failure.	Try to find the middle ground. Recognise that there is good and bad in everything and everyone. Nothing is black and white.

Extract from Monash University, Counselling and Mental Health[2]

Gratitude = the Ultimate Cure for Negative Thinking

One of the best ways I find to break negative thinking patterns is to write a gratitude list every day. By writing, say, the top five things you are grateful for in your life at the start of the day you will find that you will begin the day in a better frame of mind. After all, we have so much to be grateful for but many times we do not stop to appreciate these things.

I recall a patient of mine who found himself extremely stressed about a situation in his life. He was facing bankruptcy and kept repeating over and over, 'I'm going to lose everything.' This worry had led to anxiety, difficulty sleeping, weight loss and overwhelming fatigue. So not only was his situation not the best but it was compounded by how physically terrible he felt. When I asked him to write a list of 10 things he was still grateful for in his life it surprised him to realise that, in fact, he had not lost 'everything' but rather just lost control over 1 aspect of his life. He slowly started to gain some perspective and see that there were still things in life worth living for. There were things that were still enjoyable such as his 3 young children, his loving wife, his supportive church group, and his newfound hobby of road cycling. He realised that what he was worrying about was potential loss of material things. They were things that he had worked hard for but, ultimately, were not the things that mattered most to him. This is often the case; when writing your gratitude list, consider if you spend a lot of time worrying about things that do not really matter.

Take Home Points

Negative thinking can be habitual.

- When we think a certain way over a long period of time we develop a pattern of thinking that is either positive or negative.
- It has been suggested that negative thinking patterns can lead to a range of mental and physical health conditions due to the toxic impact of negative thoughts on the brain.
- There are some negative thought patterns that are common to everyone.
- Luckily these common negative thought patterns can be broken, with practise.
- One of the best cures for negative thinking is gratitude.
- Writing a gratitude list every morning can help set your day in a positive way.
- It is important that we learn what established patterns of negative thinking we have developed so that these can be broken before they ruin our mental and physical health.

YOUR *Weekly* CHALLENGE . . . .

This week your challenge is to identify what patterns of negative thinking you have established as a habit, either consciously or subconsciously. Consider writing a gratitude list every day of this week as a way of breaking your negative thought patterns and remembering what is really important to you in your life.

nurture yourself

Making time to nurture ourselves can often feel selfish, but self-care is so critical to mental and physical health that I would argue we perhaps should place it at the top of our priority list. This is most important when we are feeling worn out physically or mentally. It is so easy to keep going without taking stock of how we are really feeling about our lives, our health and our current relationships. But sooner or later, unless we start really nurturing ourselves, we find that we begin to resent our families, our friends, our work and our once enjoyable commitments for taking up all our time. The unfortunate result of this is frustration, fatigue, self-loathing, and a lack of overall enjoyment in our lives. The remedy to feeling this way is to realise that we are the masters of our bodies, our actions and our schedules, and to make a little time to self-nurture.

Health TIP

Just 1 hour a day of self-nurturing will make the other 23 hours of the day more productive and rewarding.

Define Your Priorities

Sometimes we feel a sense of frustration about our lives and schedules but cannot seem to place why we are feeling this way. Consider that maybe it is because we have not really considered what our priorities are.

Take a look at where most of your time is now going and think about where you would like it to be going.

Consider all of these areas of your life:

- Emotional health
- Physical health
- Relationships
- Spiritual well-being
- Work
- Service/contributions to others
- Fun/adventure/leisure

Now that you've considered these areas of your life, where would you like most of your time to be going? What areas have you neglected?

Redefining Your Time Priorities

Do you truly believe that your time is, well, exactly that? Y*our* time? What is your belief about time? Do you feel that others dictate how you spend your time? Does time feel out of your control? Here is what you need to do to begin to take control of YOUR TIME.

Get a piece of paper and make three categories across the top:

LIKE . . . . **DISLIKE** . . . . **AMBIVALENT ABOUT**

Think of a typical week in your life. Under the appropriate category, list all the activities you did during this week. For example, you might write:

LIKE	DISLIKE	AMBIVALENT ABOUT
Sleeping	Cleaning the bathtub	Watching TV
Yoga class	Mowing the lawns	Making dinner every night
Reading a good book	Paying the bills	Talking on the phone to Mum

What to Do About the Items You Dislike?

Examine the activities you listed under Dislike. Go down the list and ask yourself, 'Must I do this? And if I must, how can I change this to make it more satisfying or agreeable?'

Realise it is impossible to get rid of all the 'disliked' items on your list, but do eliminate or transform as many as you can. Be creative.

Brainstorm about how to rid yourself of these activities. Set a timer for 10 minutes and list every idea you can think of. Try to keep your hand moving. Repeat items if you need to.

Now take one action to eliminate or change a disliked activity. For example:

you could get someone else to pay the bills; you could go live in a tent by the beach so you do not have any bills to pay; you could set up direct debits so that you do not have to think about paying the bills; you could have a foot spa or neck massage while you pay your bills online ...

See? Some of the ideas are silly, some worth exploring.

What About the Ambivalent Activities?

These are probably your time devourers, simply because you are ambivalent about them. You might want to replace some of these with activities you like more.

Rescuing Time for Self-Nurturing

We all have time wasters that zap us of energy and leave us feeling frustrated. Instead of using whatever time you have left at the end of your day to spend on yourself consider using the best parts of your day when you have the most energy as your key times to do some self-care.

Consider reclaiming lost time from unnecessary activities. Here are some great ideas[1].

PHONES, COMPUTERS AND TVS

- Screen your phone calls. If you do not recognise the number let the call go to voicemail.
- If it is not a suitable time to talk say straight away, 'I'm really glad you called but I can't talk right now.' Try not to make excuses.
- Only check Facebook and emails once a day.
- Turn off the ringer.
- Choose what you watch on TV. When the program is over, immediately turn the TV off.
- Give your TV away.
- Turn off your computer at a set time every day.
- Turn off the information overload. You do not need to read every newspaper, watch the news every night or answer every email every day.

HOUSEWORK AND ERRANDS

- Let housework go. Try not to use cleaning and straightening up a room as a way to stay busy and avoid nurturing yourself.

- Enlist help. If you are married or live with someone, divide up the work. For example: you clean, do laundry and take care of the dog. Your partner can cook, shop and take out the garbage. Whatever the specifics, work it out.
- Hire a cleaning person once a month, even if you have to give something up in order to have the money to do it.
- Do not waste your peak energy times doing housework, or any other tedious work.
- Consolidate your errands by being organised so that you do 2 or more errands in one go e.g. make a shopping list so that you know exactly what you are buying.
- Complete many of your errands online such as paying bills and shopping.
- Deal with procrastination. Take 1 item at a time and just do it.
- Ask for help – you are not superhuman and others are usually glad to help.
- Finally, regularly query yourself, 'Is this how I choose to spend my time?'

After You've Freed Up Your Time, Now What?

Freeing the time and then making sure you use it for self-nurturing are two different challenges. There is a well-known rule that work expands to fill the time available. Once you make the time, you need to be sure you fill it with comforting things. This is especially true when you are trying to replace ambivalent activities with more nurturing ones.

Dream up a list of pleasurable activities you would love to do. Write this 'Nurture List' in a journal, diary or, even better, post them on the fridge so that you can be reminded to include them in your schedule regularly. Think of pleasures that encompass each area of your life:

- Physical
- Emotional
- Mental
- Spiritual

Make your list varied in terms of time requirements. That is, list activities you can do in a few minutes, an hour, a $\frac{1}{2}$ day, a day, or even 2 days.

Your list does not have to be made up entirely of solitary pleasures, but some activities you should do alone just to ensure you are basing your list on activities that you enjoy and doing things to keep someone else happy. Try to come up with at least 20 nurturing activities. This will give you variety.

Your Self-Nurture Program

Whip out your calendar and open it to tomorrow. Place your Nurture List next to your calendar. Now, on each and every day schedule 2 nurturing activities. Keep an eye out for balance. Choose activities that are realistic. For example:

MONDAY	Talk to my best friend Go for a walk
TUESDAY	Meditate for 15 minutes Watch a movie with friends
WEDNESDAY	Attend a yoga class Read for 15 minutes
THURSDAY	Go to the library and find books on things that interest me. Get a massage.
FRIDAY	Put on music and do spontaneous exercise for 20 minutes. Have a nice dinner with my lover.

Take Home Points

- Self-nurturing is key to maintaining a balanced approach to health, work and relationships.
- Self-nurturing is not selfish but a necessity.
- The key to self-nurturing is recognising your priorities.
- Waiting until you are less busy to start self-nurturing means that realistically it will never happen.
- We have to prioritise self-nurturing in our schedules each week.
- Waiting until we are worn out to begin self-nurturing means we have waited too long.
- Thinking of self-nurturing activities that you enjoy, ahead of time, is a great way to make sure that you do not forget to include them in your busy weekly schedule.
- Self-nurturing does not need to be exclusionary and can, of course, include the company of those you love.

YOUR *Weekly* CHALLENGE · · · · · · · · · · · ·

This week your challenge is to make a list of at least 20 nurturing activities that you can include in your schedule. Make sure you prioritise these in your diary and see how much more energised and less frustrated you feel at the end of the week for doing so.

have a
health check

Modern medicine has come such a long way. We have a range of screening tests available to us that detect various health conditions. Many of these screening tests are relatively non-invasive, inexpensive and easy to do. With this in mind it surprises me that the current statistics show that only $\frac{2}{3}$ of eligible Australian women undertake the recommended Pap testing and mammogram[1]. Similarly, just over $\frac{1}{3}$ of Australian men and women undertake the recommended bowel cancer screening[2]. I highly recommend all adults undertake the recommended health checks. These may just save your life if a potentially fatal health condition is detected early enough to treat.

What Exactly Are Health Checks?

Health checks are done by a doctor, usually a general practitioner or family physician, to detect any common, treatable or potentially serious health conditions. Getting a health check is important for all Australian adults as some health conditions have only mild or no symptoms, which means that even though you are feeling well you still may be harbouring a serious disease.

How Often Should You Have a Health Check?

I recommend all Australian adults have a health check at least every second year from the age of 18 years. A health check may comprise of the some of following depending on whether you have any symptoms, your past medical history and your family medical history:

- **Blood pressure screening**
- **Blood testing** To look for nutritional deficiencies, hormone imbalances, thyroid conditions, liver and kidney conditions, high cholesterol and diabetes.
- **Cancer screening** For example, skin checks to detect skin cancers, Pap tests every 2 years for women to detect cervical cancer, breast examinations at any age for

women as well as a mammogram in those older than 40 years to detect breast cancer, bowel cancer screening, and prostate and testicular cancer screening for men.

- **Heart screening** This might include an electrocardiogram (ECG) to check your heart rhythm and heart health. This might also include a referral for an exercise stress test to ensure you are not at risk of a heart attack.

- **Lung screening** This might include a spirometry lung function test to rule out asthma and/or other lung conditions. It may also include a referral for a chest X-ray, especially in smokers, to rule out cancer or other conditions.

- **Eye screening** Traditionally undertaken by an optometrist to check eye health.

- **Genetic screening** There are situations where genetic screening is undertaken to determine your genetic risk for a disease. This is often done in consultation with a genetic counsellor, especially where the condition has serious implications for your health or that of your family.

Health FACT . . . .

Conditions such as high blood pressure, diabetes and high cholesterol often have no symptoms. That is why they are known as the 'silent killers'.

Where Do You Go to Get A Health Check?

Your local general practitioner is the best person to see to organise having a comprehensive health check. In some cities there are also specialised women's and men's health clinics that undertake health screening. If you have already had a recent health check but find that you have one or more of the health warning signs listed on page 163 consult with your health practitioner sooner rather than later. It is better to be safe than sorry when it comes to health warning signs. As a doctor I have seen the devastating consequences when someone exhibiting significant health warning signs puts off seeing me until it is too late.

Will A Health Check Be Painful?

Many people feel uncomfortable seeing a doctor sometimes due to negative past experiences or because they are afraid of what the doctor may or may not find. Consider that doctors are human too and in general we want to be compassionate about your situation and your health concerns. We do not like to inflict unnecessary discomfort, embarrassment, or unease. Unfortunately, though, sometimes having to undertake necessary health checks can be uncomfortable, albeit tolerable. In reality, we are so fortunate to be given access to inexpensive, high quality medical care. There are many individuals in less opportune circumstances who would greatly appreciate equivalent care. Perhaps keeping this in mind will help us to take the steps needed to make sure our health is in check. We really do owe it to ourselves and our families.

Watch Out for Health Warning Signs

Basically, if you notice anything unusual in your body or you are concerned about anything go and see your health practitioner for their advice. Try to avoid the temptation to consult 'Doctor Google'. More often than not you will end up confused and unnecessarily concerned by what you read on the internet. Your health practitioner is the best person to diagnose your health condition. If you feel that symptoms persist despite advice you have been given, please go back and see your health practitioner again. They will no doubt undertake further investigations to uncover the root cause. If you still feel that symptoms persist seek a second opinion. There is no harm in doing so and, as a health practitioner myself, I can honestly say we are not offended by this.

There are some common health warning signs to look out for and these include:

- Sweating for no reason at night time
- Losing weight for no reason
- Unexplained easy bruising
- Chest pains or discomfort, especially pain that radiates to your jaw or down your left arm
- Any unexplained vaginal or rectal bleeding
- Constant fatigue
- Feelings of consistently low mood or suicidal thoughts
- Difficulty breathing
- Coughing, vomiting or urinating blood
- A lump that you have discovered
- A new mole or freckle or a change in an existing mole or freckle
- Recurrent infections
- Severe, consistent or recurrent pain anywhere in your body
- Difficulty sleeping

If you have any of these symptoms do consult with your health practitioner as soon as possible. Although relatively benign conditions can also present with the above signs and symptoms they can also be an indication of something more serious.

Take Home Points

Having a health check may save your life.

- There are effective and safe screening tests available for many common and/or serious health conditions.
- I recommend all adults undertake at least second-yearly health screening with their local general practitioner or family physician.
- Although seeing your doctor for a health check may be slightly uncomfortable, potentially even a little embarrassing and may bring with it some anxiety, it is well worth the short period of unease for the benefit of safeguarding your health.
- Health warning signs should not be ignored. Seeing your health care practitioner immediately is advised if you are concerned about any symptoms or signs that you may be experiencing.

YOUR *Weekly* CHALLENGE . . . .

This week your challenge is to have a health check by your general practitioner if you have not had one for several years or if you are experiencing any concerning signs and symptoms.

move more

Our bodies were made to move. With over 200 bones in our bodies, 650 muscles, and 360 joints working as levers to create movement it is clear that we are designed to be active. There are so many health benefits to exercise. If there is one thing you could start doing today to greatly improve your health it would be to move more. With the way society is today, with the majority of us holding sedentary jobs, we have to make a little effort when it comes to getting enough exercise. In times gone by most of the exercise we did would be incidental in the form of manual labour and/or tending to our home, yard and small children. There were no gyms until the early 1980s. Most of us did not need the extra exercise.

But of course times have changed and fewer and fewer of us are getting the recommended amount of exercise per week. Studies show that only around $\frac{1}{3}$ of Australians undertake regular physical activity, with women being less active on average than men[1]. Considering the health benefits of exercise we really do need to learn to incorporate it into our lifestyles as a lifelong habit. So what are the health benefits of exercise? What is the best type of exercise to do and how long do you need to exercise for to reap the benefits?

Health FACT
Physical inactivity is the 4th leading cause of death due to chronic disease worldwide – contributing to over 3 million preventable deaths annually[2].

How to Stay Motivated

It is not uncommon for people to embark upon a new exercise regimen with plenty of enthusiasm only to give up after a few weeks. Here are some ways to maintain motivation so that you can continue exercising.

These include:

- Find an activity you enjoy – this is key to sustainability.

- Create non-food rewards. Once you reach your health goals reward yourself with something that is not food-based e.g. go to the cinema, have a massage, buy yourself a new outfit, or even reward yourself with a holiday.

- Create accountability. Wherever possible make sure you are accountable to someone else with your health goals. This may involve, for example, finding a training partner or just sticking your health goals on the fridge so that your family is aware of them and can help keep you on track.

- Use gadgets e.g. pedometer, heart-rate monitor. These help to gauge your progress and keep your training measurable and objective.

- Set goals. Keep in mind that if you aim at nothing you are sure to hit it. Writing down your health goals for the year helps your subconscious mind to work towards these. When you write down a goal also write down your reason for wanting to achieve this goal. Make it a compelling reason, which will help to keep you motivated when you feel like giving up, such as, 'I want to be fit so that I can have the stamina to play with my kids (or grandkids) after work'.

- Create a fail-safe routine. By this I mean make sure there is no reason why you could bail on your exercise and health routine. An example might be setting up your gym clothes the night beforehand at the end of your bed. When you wake up in the morning you cannot use the excuse that you are not prepared and have nothing to wear.

- Choose an activity that doesn't involve a lot of travel and suits your budget. You should not have to drive for hours on end or spend a fortune on your exercise routine. Going for a brisk walk or jog around the block can be just as effective as any other exercise.

- Don't think too much about it. If you are spending precious time trying to plan the best type of exercise, the best gym to go to, and the perfect outfit, then chances are it will all start to 'get too hard'. To quote the famous Nike slogan, 'Just Do It'.

Next we will debunk some exercise myths that I commonly hear so that we can eliminate any barriers for not exercising.

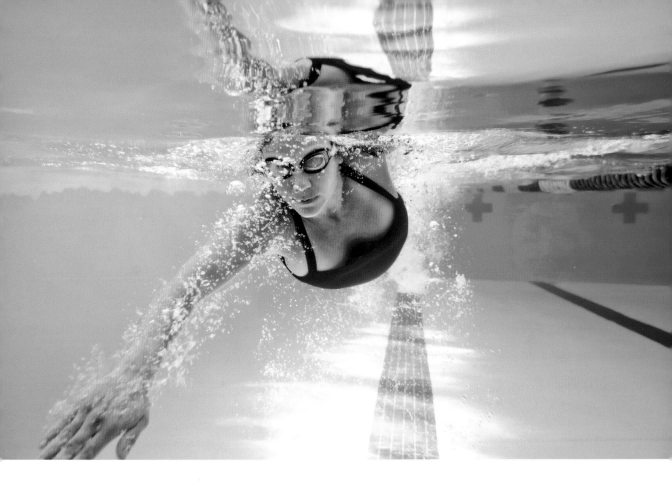

Common Exercise Myths Debunked

Myth Number 1: I'm tired already; won't exercise make me even more tired? Studies indicate that regular exercise actually increases your energy. You have to use energy to create energy. The body works in equilibrium and in balance – if you use less energy, your body will not need to produce as much.

Myth Number 2: But I'm in too much pain to exercise. Although you may indeed be in a lot of pain, exercise actually reduces pain levels over time. It causes release of our body's own natural painkillers, known as endorphins and leads to conditioning of the body to resist pain.

Myth Number 3: It's all too complicated, and I really don't like going to the gym. Just do something that you enjoy. Exercise is simply any movement that causes us to sweat and increases our heart rate. Start with walking, which is really one of the best exercises we can do. It is low-impact on the joints and can help us lose weight. For example, adding 30 mins of brisk walking 4 times per week will mean you could lose up to 15 per cent of your body weight per year without even changing your diet.

Myth Number 4: I really don't have the time to commit to an exercise program right now. It does not take a lot of effort to start realising the health benefits of exercise. Just start with 5 minutes per day 3 or 4 times per week, and build up to 30 minutes per day most days of the week. Remember, as with most important things in our life, we have to make the time for them rather than wait for an opportunity to arise in our schedules.

Myth Number 5: I want to lose weight off my tummy and thighs, so shouldn't I just be concentrating on those areas alone? Although toning exercises may strengthen and tighten the muscle underneath the layer of fat that overlies that muscle, we may not actually see a change in size of our tummy or thighs. This is because to lose the fat overlying the muscle, we need to burn it off. This can only be achieved by elevating our heart rate and using energy. Many toning exercises do not work our body enough to sweat and burn fat. The best fat burning exercises are aerobic exercises like brisk walking, swimming, jogging or bike riding.

Take Home Points

Many of us are not getting enough exercise.

- This is contributing to the many health problems that doctors see nowadays, including obesity, heart disease, diabetes, strokes, arthritis and vitamin D deficiency.
- Making exercise a lifelong habit will help to ensure good health.
- It is important that we make exercising a priority.
- Just 30 minutes a day most days a week will have a significant impact on our health and well-being.
- Alternate your training schedule to incorporate some cardiovascular exercise ('huffy puffy'), resistance training, as well as flexibility and core strength training as these all have different and equally important benefits.
- To keep motivated find an activity you enjoy, create some accountability, set achievable goals, reward yourself regularly, and keep the attitude of 'just do it' rather than making excuses.

YOUR *Weekly* CHALLENGE . . . .

This week your challenge is to make the time to exercise. If you are not used to exercising start slow and build up. Find an activity you enjoy and consider enlisting the support of a family member or friend as your training partner.

avoid injury

Sporting and exercise injuries are common but can largely be prevented. Too often I see newly motivated individuals start an exercise programme and shortly afterwards develop an injury. This can often be a disappointing setback and can even cause people to be too scared to exercise. But injuries associated with exercise and sports need not occur if we follow some of the simple tips below.

Health FACT . . . .

Exercise injuries may be prevented by properly warming up and cooling down, wearing quality footwear and doing gentle stretching.

Top 5 Tips to Avoid Injury

The following tips may seem intuitive but can be helpful in reducing injury rate from exercising in general. Keep in mind that this list is not all inclusive. If you do experience an injury or have noticed that you are injury prone in a particular area of your body then do seek professional advice from your local physiotherapist (physical therapist) before embarking on any strenuous exercise program.

TIP #1 START SLOW

Starting out exercising like a bull at a gate is all well and good until we get hurt. Consider that a more sensible approach is to build up your exercise tolerance and fitness slowly. If you are not used to exercising at all or have not exercised in quite a while consider starting with gentle exercises such as walking, swimming or bike riding. Once you have mastered a certain level of fitness consider increasing the duration and/or intensity of the exercise.

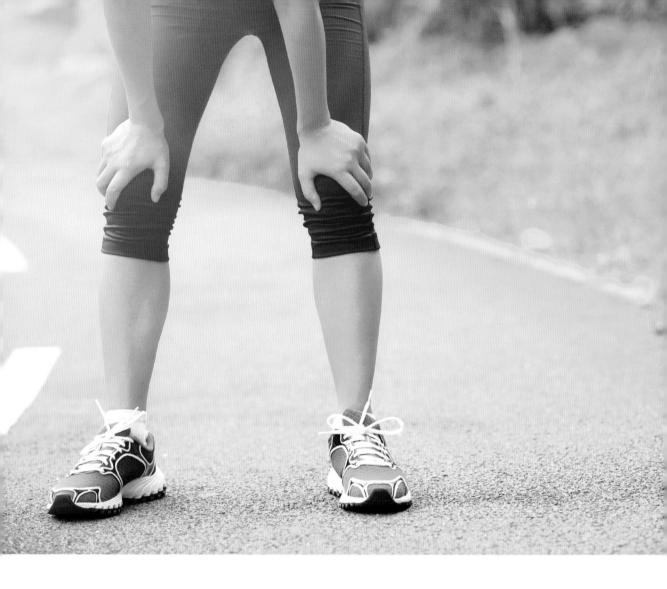

Keep in mind that if you have not exercised for a long time or you undertake a new exercise you may experience some delayed-onset muscle soreness (DOMS), which is normal and usually resolves within a few days. If this is excessively painful or debilitating next time you exercise reduce the intensity and time that you exercise for and increase more slowly. Having an Epsom salts bath, drinking plenty of water, resting, and having a light massage can be helpful to recover quicker from exercise.

Note too that if you are experiencing chest pains, excessive shortness of breath, dizziness, blurred vision, or any other unusual sensations then stop exercising immediately and seek medical attention before exercising again. These are all warning signs that something more serious may be going on. Consider too that exercise should not be excessively painful. If something hurts then stop and seek professional advice to find out what might be causing you to have pain.

TIP #2 WEAR QUALITY SHOES

Quality footwear is important to prevent foot, ankle, knee, hip and back injuries. Wearing worn out sneakers with very little support is potentially going to leave your body very sore. Consider purchasing some quality sneakers that offer the correct amount of support for your foot. The best approach would be to seek advice from those trained in footwear and foot positioning. Your local physiotherapist or podiatrist would be able to assist with this. Occasionally orthotics need to be inserted into footwear to offer additional support. This is particularly the case if your foot rolls in or out or you suffer any pains in your feet/ankles when exercising. Once again your local physiotherapist or podiatrist will be able to assist with this.

TIP #3 KNOW YOUR BODY TYPE

My husband, who is a physiotherapist and author of the book *You Can Run Pain Free: A Physio's 5 Step Guide to Enjoying Injury-Free and Faster Running* often refers to the comical yet descriptive terms 'flippy', 'floppy' or 'stiffy' to describe the three most common body types when it comes to ligament stability and flexibility, and therefore susceptibility to injury[1].

He states that floppy individuals are those who are hypermobile and can be prone to joint injuries due to the fact that their joints are not well protected by stable ligaments. You know you are a floppy if you are 'double-jointed' i.e. if you are able to bend your thumb downwards to touch your wrist. These individuals benefit from a balanced strength-training program to develop the muscles around their joints to prevent injuries. The next individuals who can be prone to injuries are the stiffy group. These individuals find flexibility exercises difficult and benefit from gentle stretching exercises to improve their overall flexibility and fluidity of body movements to prevent injury. The flippy individuals are in between these two types and are neither hypermobile nor very stiff. These individuals are less prone to injuries than the floppy and stiffy group. However, they still benefit from a guided strength and flexibility program.

Knowing what body type you are can help to avoid injury. The better approach would be to seek a trained physiotherapist if you find yourself prone to injuries or better still before you begin an exercise program to make sure that you prevent injuries from occurring.

TIP #4 WARM UP & COOL DOWN

There is some evidence to suggest that warming up for 5–10 minutes before exercise may help to reduce injury rates. This may involve brisk walking: for example, before going for your jog. Much like a manual car that needs to go through each gear sequentially it makes sense to warm up the body by slowly increasing your intensity of exercise up to your maximal effort.

Similarly, cooling down after exercise for 5-10 minutes may help to prevent injuries from occurring. This also may help lactic acid to dissipate from muscles, preventing muscle soreness. Keep in mind that muscle soreness (DOMS) is common 48 hours following exercise. This does not mean you have had an injury but that the muscles are repairing and adapting to the exercise. During this time gentle exercise, cold/heat packs, magnesium supplements and light massage may help relieve the pains.

TIP #5 STRETCH

Stretching following exercise whilst your muscles are still warm may help to prevent injury and alleviate muscle soreness. Never stretch to the point of excessive pain. Just a gentle pull should be experienced. Avoid stretching that involves hyperextending the spine forwards or backwards and avoid bouncing whilst stretching. Simply holding a static stretch for 1-2 minutes each side is enough.

Hopefully these tips will help us to remain injury free and keep us exercising well into our older years without any debilitating aches and pains.

Take Home Points

Injuries and exercise should not go hand in hand.

- We can hopefully avoid injury by gently warming up and cooling down after exercise, by wearing quality shoes, and by gently stretching. Knowing our body types when it comes to our joint stability and flexibility may also help us to avoid injury.
- Anytime we experience warning signs while exercising, such as shortness of breath, chest pains, dizziness or blurred vision, we should stop exercising immediately and seek medical attention.
- Keep in mind that exercise should be enjoyable and not excessively painful.

YOUR *Weekly* CHALLENGE . . . .

This week your challenge is to avoid injury whilst exercising by purchasing quality footwear, remembering to warm up and cool down before and after exercise, and by doing some gentle stretching following exercise.

look after your posture

Interestingly many of our aches and pains are due to our poor postures. Going back 100 years this was not as much of an issue as it is now – with many of us stooped over a desk for most of the day. Even our kids are developing postural issues due to having less playtime and needing more study time to keep up with today's gruelling curriculum. So how do we look after our posture to avoid the common muscular and skeletal conditions that can come from not having our spine correctly aligned?

Health FACT . . . .

Neck and back pain can largely be prevented by correcting our posture.

What Are The Symptoms of Poor Posture?

When you compare the pictures on page 177 of correct and poor posture, you can quickly see why the following symptoms of poor posture can arise.

   I learnt this first hand as I suffered for quite a few years from neck pain to the point that I thought that I would one day need to have surgery. I was getting shooting pains down my arms especially at night. I noticed that these symptoms would all get worse around university exam time and when I was stressed. But I did not correlate my symptoms with my poor studying posture. I had a bad habit of stooping over my text books for many hours at a time without having a break. To make matters worse others had started noticing my slouched posture. My family would say to me, 'Stand up straight.' Luckily I married a physiotherapist (physical therapist) and quickly learnt from him all about correct posture and why this is so important. To this day I am very mindful of my posture and do all that I can to look after it. I am pleased to report that I am pain free more days than not and the shooting pains have stopped. But you don't need to marry a physio to know when you might need to change your posture. These symptoms may be a sign that you are in need of some guidance in this area:

- Stiff neck muscles
- Difficulty turning your head either with or without pain
- Headaches
- Tight upper back muscles
- Back stiffness and pain
- Pinched nerves in your spine
- Lower back pain
- Tender spots or 'knots' in your back or neck muscles

These symptoms occur because the smaller supportive central muscles that hold up our spine become weakened and/or fatigued due to poor spinal alignment. The larger muscles are then forced to do the job of the smaller spinal support muscles and become tight as a result. The outcome is taut, tender muscles. The worst outcome in this situation is that if our posture remains poorly aligned for too long we can develop permanent skeletal changes such as a curved spine (scoliosis), a humpback (kyphosis), and/or a sway back (lordosis). Fortunately these conditions can be largely prevented; even if we were born with some skeletal misalignments, they can be improved and prevented from worsening with correct postural techniques.

How Can You Look After Your Posture?

The first step in looking after our posture is to learn how to stand and sit correctly. These basics are explained below.

CORRECT STANDING

When we stand we should aim to have our weight evenly distributed between both feet with our centre of gravity at the middle of each foot. Do not lock your knees but have them slightly bent. Our ears should line up with our shoulders, and our shoulders should line up with our hips. Think tall, slightly puff out your chest, tuck your chin in, and slightly tuck your bottom under. Just by doing that you will feel better. To remind yourself to stand correctly, consider putting a small sticker on your watch, mobile or other device that you check regularly. Every time you see that sticker you will be prompted to stand tall again. Practice makes perfect and as your spinal, postural muscles strengthen you will find yourself standing tall without having to think about it.

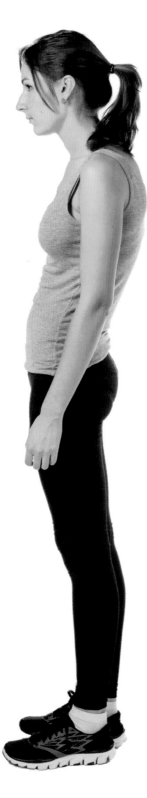
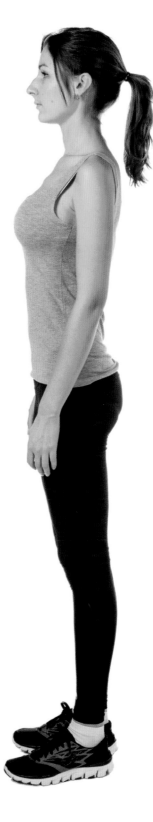

Poor Posture
v Correct Posture

CORRECT SITTING

When we are sitting it is easy to slouch over our computer or desk. This leaves us open to lower back and neck pain. To correct this, sit up tall in your chair. Make sure both your feet can touch the floor and that your bottom is well back in the chair. Maintain the normal curvature of the lower spine by rolling up a small towel to place in the small of your back, or purchase a lumbar support. Your chair should be positioned vertically so that your knees are slightly lower than your hips. You should be able to see your computer at eye level easily and have your forearms resting on the desk. Elevating your laptop screen with a few books placed underneath may help correctly position the screen to eye level. Remember to have regular breaks from typing and stand up, stretch slightly and then sit back down.

If you are still having ongoing problems with neck or back pain seeing your local physiotherapist (physical therapist) is recommended. Physiotherapists are health professionals who are trained to show you the correct way to align your posture, ease your aches and pains, and help you strengthen your postural muscles to prevent any problems arising from poor posture.

Take Home Points

Correct posture is important to prevent neck and back pains as well as skeletal problems.

- Many of us have poor posture due to our modern-day lifestyles with more screen time than ever.
- We may need to constantly remind ourselves about correct posture when we stand and sit and a useful way might be to place a sticker in the corner of our computer screens, phones or watches. Every time we see that sticker we will be reminded to stand and sit up straighter.
- Practice makes perfect and as our postural spinal muscles become stronger and our spine becomes more consistently aligned we will find ourselves automatically standing and sitting with correct posture.

YOUR *Weekly* CHALLENGE . . . .

This week your challenge is to stand and sit tall. Look at the images of what correct posture for standing entails and try and replicate this throughout your day. The result will be less muscular pains and fatigue.

protect your pelvic floor

Many of us have heard the term pelvic floor before but few of us really know where it is and how important it is to our sexual and urological health. I have met numerous patients who have experienced a level of pelvic floor dysfunction and many people endure this condition for many years. It has become so commonplace to them that they do not realise that there are effective treatment options available so that they do not have to put up with the embarrassing and/or painful symptoms any longer. It is astounding when you realise how many of us experience the symptoms of pelvic floor dysfunction.

Health FACT . . . .

Urinary incontinence is a sign of pelvic floor weakness and affects up to 13 per cent of men and up to 37 per cent of women in Australia[1].

What Is the Pelvic Floor?

The pelvic floor is a layer of muscles that supports the pelvic organs and spans the bottom of the pelvis. The pelvic organs are the bladder and bowel in men, and bladder, bowel and uterus in women. The diagrams on page 180 shows the pelvic organs and pelvic floor muscles in women (right) and men (left).

As indicated in the diagram, the pelvic floor muscles stretch from the tailbone (coccyx) to the pubic bone (front to back) and from one sitting bone to the other sitting bone (side to side). These muscles are normally firm and thick.

Imagine the pelvic floor muscles as a round mini-trampoline made of firm muscle. Just like a trampoline, the pelvic floor is able to move down and up. The bladder, uterus (for women) and bowel lie on the pelvic floor muscle layer.

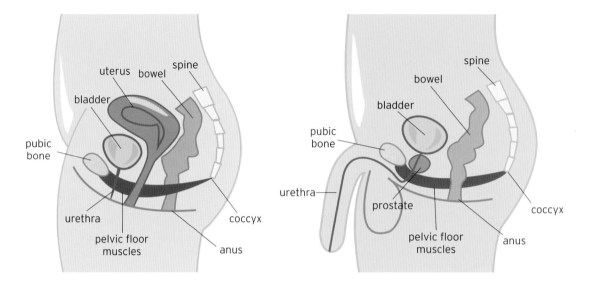

The pelvic floor muscle layer has holes for passages to pass through. There are two passages in men (the urethra and anus) and three passages in women (the urethra, vagina and anus). The pelvic floor muscles normally wrap quite firmly around these holes to help keep the passages shut except when in use. There is also an extra, circular muscle around the anus (the anal sphincter) and around the urethra (the urethral sphincter).

What do Pelvic Floor Muscles Do?

Pelvic floor muscles provide support to the organs that lie on it. The sphincters give us conscious control over the bladder and bowel so that we can control the release of urine, faeces and wind, and allow us to delay emptying until it is convenient. When the pelvic floor muscles are contracted, the internal organs are lifted and the sphincters tighten the openings of the vagina, anus and urethra. Relaxing the pelvic floor allows passage of urine, wind and faeces.

Pelvic floor muscles are also important for sexual function in both men and women. In men, it is important for erectile function and ejaculation. In women, voluntary contractions (squeezing) of the pelvic floor contribute to sexual sensation and arousal.

The pelvic floor muscles in women also provide support for the baby during pregnancy and assist in the birthing process.

The muscles of the pelvic floor work with the abdominal and back muscles to stabilise and support the spine (more on this in the next chapter).

Signs that You May Have a Pelvic Floor Problem

Common signs that can indicate a pelvic floor problem include:

• Accidentally leaking urine when you exercise, laugh, cough or sneeze

- Needing to get to the toilet in a hurry or not making it there in time
- Constantly needing to go to the toilet
- Finding it difficult to empty your bladder or bowel
- Accidentally losing control of your bladder or bowel
- Accidentally passing wind
- A prolapse - in women, this may be felt as a bulge in the vagina or a feeling of heaviness, discomfort, pulling, dragging or dropping. In men this may be felt as a bulge in the rectum or a feeling of needing to use their bowels but not actually needing to go
- Pain in your pelvic area
- Painful sex.

What Can Cause Pelvic Floor Problems?

Pelvic floor problems can occur when the pelvic floor muscles are stretched, weakened or too tight. Some people have weak pelvic floor muscles from an early age, while others notice problems after certain life stages such as pregnancy, childbirth or menopause. On the other hand, some people have pelvic floor muscles that are too tight and cannot relax. This can be made worse by doing squeezing exercises and overworking the muscles without learning how to relax.

Pelvic floor muscle fitness is affected by a number of things, including:

- Not keeping your pelvic floor active (more on strengthening your pelvic floor in the next chapter)
- Being pregnant and having babies
- A history of back pain
- Ongoing constipation and straining to empty the bowels
- Carrying too much weight for your frame
- Heavy lifting
- A chronic cough or sneeze, including those who have asthma, those who smoke or suffer from hay fever
- Previous injury to the pelvic region (e.g. a fall or surgery)
- Hormone changes in menopause
- General ageing process

What Can You Do to Protect Your Pelvic Floor?

The following principles will help prevent damage to your pelvic floor:

Avoid heavy lifting This can create pressure on the pelvic floor and ultimately lead to prolapse. Men and women in certain professions - such as nursing or courier services, for example - are at particular risk. People performing heavy weight training at a gym

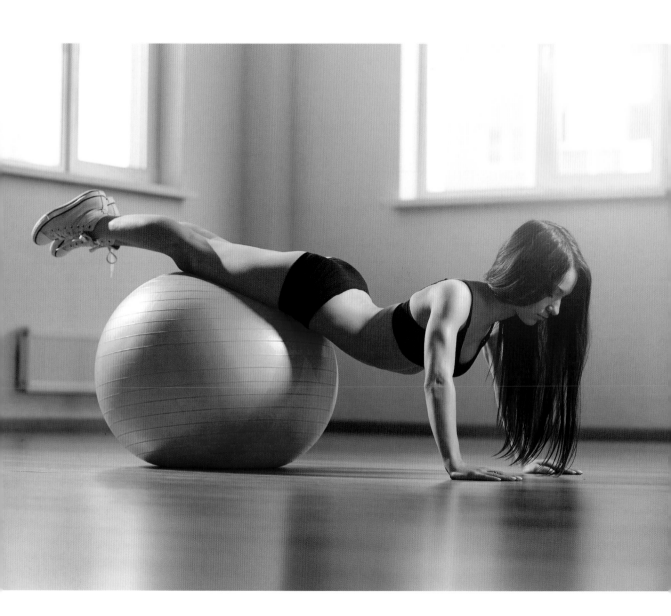

can also be at risk of straining the pelvic floor. Whenever you are lifting something heavy, maintain good posture, bend from the knees and not from the hips, and exhale when you lift rather than hold your breath.

When exercising adopt supported positions – sitting on a fit ball, lying on a bench, or resting against a wall will help to protect your pelvic floor from overstraining. Try keeping your feet closer together with certain exercises such as squats as this will help to activate your pelvic floor more easily. Avoid exercising when you are tired and try to break between sets for a few minutes to give your pelvic floor a rest. If you have pelvic floor problems, you must keep your resistance to a minimum until your pelvic floor muscle condition has improved. Avoid lifting weights from ground level if possible; instead, aim to lift from waist height.

Avoid high impact exercises This includes running, basketball, netball and aerobics classes. If you enjoy participating in these types of sports try to mix them up with other types of pelvic-floor safe exercises such as swimming, walking, cycling, yoga and Pilates so that you are not putting strain on the pelvic floor all the time.

Be careful with pregnancy Pelvic floor weakness can begin in pregnancy due to the effects of certain hormones released in pregnancy that loosen ligaments as well as the extra weight that is gained. A prolonged or difficult labour, a large baby, and an instrumental delivery (forceps or vacuum extraction) can further weaken the pelvic floor. Pelvic floor damage can be accelerated, however, if women return to heavy lifting or high impact sport either during pregnancy or too soon after the delivery of their baby. I have even heard it quoted that the pelvic floor remains vulnerable to increased levels of damage up to 3 months after a woman stops breastfeeding. The best approach is gentle exercises such as walking, swimming, cycling and gentle stretching.

Deal with chronic coughing If you have been coughing either consistently or intermittently over the years then this could be gradually weakening your pelvic floor. Chronic coughing can be caused by asthma, smoking, acid reflux, and other rarer medical conditions. Discuss your chronic cough with your doctor who will be able to help treat the cause.

Avoid constipation Chronic straining whilst on the toilet can lead to pelvic floor weakness and/or prolapse of the organs into the vagina (for women) or the anus (the rectal lining protrudes from the anus). It is important to address the cause of any constipation and learn correct toilet posture (see point below).

Practise correct toilet posture When you sit on the toilet have your elbows on knees, lean forward and support your feet with a footstool. This helps to fully relax your pelvic floor and sphincter muscles. Bulge out your tummy, relax your back passage and let go (don't hold your breath or strain). When you have finished firmly draw up your back passage.

How Can Pelvic Floor Problems Be Diagnosed?

Pelvic floor issues can be diagnosed by a pelvic floor physiotherapist, who may perform an internal examination and/or ultrasound. If your pelvic floor issue is quite severe then you may be referred to a urogynaecologist for further assessment.

Where Can You Go For Further Help?

The best first point of referral for a pelvic floor issue is your local doctor and/or a physiotherapist trained in pelvic floor management. Often pelvic floor issues can be greatly improved by learning how to strengthen your core (more on this in the next chapter).

Take Home Points

Pelvic floor issues are very common.

- The pelvic floor is a layer of muscles that lie at the base of the pelvis to support the pelvic organs.
- The pelvic floor can be weakened by repeated heavy lifting, high-impact exercises and activities, pregnancy and childbirth, chronic coughing, as well as by the general ageing process.
- When there is weakness of the pelvic floor you can experience problems with urinary and/or faecal incontinence, difficulty going to the toilet, as well as sexual health issues.
- Tightness of the pelvic floor and inability to relax can cause urinary urgency, needing to go to the toilet all the time, as well as painful sex.
- It is important to protect your pelvic floor to prevent further damage.
- A trained pelvic floor physiotherapist can help diagnose the extent of your pelvic floor issues as well as provide exercises to improve your pelvic floor strength.

YOUR *Weekly* CHALLENGE . . . .

This week your challenge is to protect your pelvic floor by following the suggestions in this chapter. If you suspect that you may have pelvic floor issues consider seeking further medical advice from your doctor or a physiotherapist trained in pelvic floor management.

strengthen your core

We have all heard it said how important it is to strengthen our core yet few people really know what this means. Core muscle strength is important to maintain correct posture and stabilise the spine to allow ease of movement, help protect the pelvic organs from prolapse, maintain sexual function, and prevent lower back pain. Core muscle training is often neglected in preference for working larger muscles since our core muscles are deep and invisible to the eye and the benefits are not often seen.

So what exactly are we referring to when we talk about our core and how can we go about safely exercising it?

Health FACT

The core forms a supportive central link between your upper and lower body. Much like a tree trunk, core muscles need to be strong yet flexible[1].

So What Exactly is Your Core?

Our core muscles include our pelvic floor as well as our deep back and abdominal muscles. These work with our diaphragm to support our spine and control the pressure within our abdomen.

During exercise, lifting, bending and twisting, the internal pressure in the abdomen changes. For example, when lifting something heavy the internal pressure increases, when we put that object down the internal pressure returns to normal.

Ideally the regulation of pressure within the abdomen happens automatically. For example, when lifting up an object, the muscles of the 'core' work together well - the pelvic floor muscles lift, the abdominal and back muscles draw in to support the spine, and breathing is easy (Diagram 1). In this scenario, the pelvic floor muscles respond appropriately to the increase in abdominal pressure.

If any of the muscles of the 'core', including the pelvic floor, are weakened or damaged, this coordinated automatic action may be altered. In this situation, during activities that increase the internal abdominal pressure, there is potential to overload the pelvic floor (Diagram 2) and/or cause lower back strain. A weakened core can lead to other injuries due to the fact that it does not have the strength to maintain correct posture and muscle positioning during movements and activities.

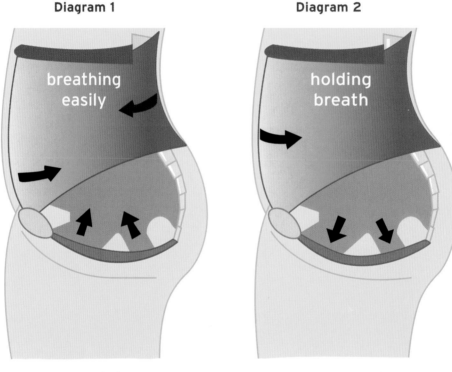

Diagram 1

breathing easily

Diagram 2

holding breath

CORRECT ACTION
The Pelvic floor lifts, the deep
abdominals draw in and
there is no change in breathing

INCORRECT ACTION
Pulling the belly button in towards
the backbone and holding your breath
can cause bearing-down on pelvic floor

How to Strengthen Your Core

The key to successfully strengthening your core is to start slowly with simple exercises, build up repetitions as your strength improves, and listen to your fatigue levels. If you are becoming tired or feel a little worn out before exercising be kind to your body and listen to these cues. Pushing past this point may lead to injury.

Some examples of exercises that strengthen the core but are safe for the pelvic floor include:

- Knees side to side with feet on ball
- Modified plank on hands or knees with a slight bend at the hips
- Wall push-ups
- Ball bridge (feet on ball or back on ball, single leg lift)
- Opposite arm and leg lift on all fours
- Leg lift sitting on the ball
- shoulder rotations with back on the ball
- Standing balance work on a bosu or balance disc

Core exercises to avoid if you have pelvic floor weakness or lower back pain:

- Sit-ups, curl-ups or crunches
- Abdominal exercises with a medicine ball
- Deep squats or lunges
- Double leg lowers
- Plank position on hands and feet (e.g. 'hovers')

Other exercises to include regularly in your daily routine are simple pelvic floor exercises. These can be done whilst driving in the car, sitting at your desk, standing in line at the supermarket, or whilst you are lying down watching television at night. Done frequently enough these exercises will help to keep the pelvic floor muscles toned.

Before starting a pelvic floor muscle training program it is important that you can identify your pelvic floor muscles correctly.

Identifying Your Pelvic Floor

The first step in performing pelvic floor muscle exercises is to identify the correct muscles. There are a couple of ways to do this:

Method 1: Stopping the flow Try to stop or slow the flow of urine midway through emptying the bladder. Stopping the flow of urine repeatedly on the toilet is not an exercise, but a way of identifying your pelvic floor muscles. This should only be done to identify which muscles are needed for bladder control as it can lead to bladder urgency. If you can, stop the flow of urine over the toilet for a second or two, then relax and finish emptying without straining. This 'stop-test' may help you identify the muscles around the front passage, which control the flow of urine.

Method 2: Visualisation Imagine stopping the flow of urine and holding in wind at the same time. This can be done lying down, sitting or standing with legs about shoulder width apart.

- Relax the muscles of your thighs, bottom and tummy.
- Squeeze in the muscles around the front passage as if trying to stop the flow of urine.
- Squeeze in the muscles around the vagina or scrotum and suck upwards inside the pelvis.
- Squeeze in the muscles around the back passage as if trying to stop passing wind.
- The muscles around the front and back passages should squeeze up and inside the pelvis.
- Identify the muscles that contract when you do all these things together. Then relax and loosen them.

Exercising Your Pelvic Floor

If you have mastered the art of contracting your pelvic floor muscles correctly, you can try holding the inward squeeze for longer (up to 10 seconds) before relaxing. Make sure you can breathe easily while you squeeze.

If you can do this exercise, repeat it up to 10 times, but only as long as you can do it with good technique while breathing quietly and keeping everything above the belly button relaxed. This can be done more often during the day to improve control.

If you go to the gym, try this exercise while lifting weights (standing) and relax fully between sets or repetitions. The goal is for your pelvic floor to be working immediately before and as you lift/lower/push or pull any load.

When to Seek Professional Help

Seek professional help from either your doctor or a physiotherapist if you have any of the symptoms below:

- Deep pain in your abdominals or back
- Pain with lifting, bending, twisting or standing
- Needing to urgently or frequently go to the toilet to pass urine or bowel motions
- Accidental leakage of urine, bowel motions or wind
- Difficulty emptying your bladder or bowel
- Vaginal heaviness or a bulge
- Pain in the bladder, bowel or in your back near the pelvic floor area when exercising the pelvic floor or during intercourse

Take Home Points

Our core is the supportive muscle structure that lie deep in our trunk.

- These muscles protect our internal organs from changes in pressure as well as supporting our spine during body movements.
- A weakened core can lead to back pain, prolapse, incontinence issues, sexual dysfunction, as well as other injuries due to lack of stabilisation.
- It is important that we protect our pelvic floor from damage when we exercise our core as well as when we exercise our larger muscles.
- Core exercises that are safe for the pelvic floor are those that are supported by the floor, a wall, a fit ball or a bench. Keep in mind to maintain good posture at all times when performing any exercises.
- Avoid abdominal crunches, deep lunges and squats, as well as any exercises that put strain on your lower back.
- It is important that we regularly perform pelvic floor exercises.
- Stopping the flow of urine and visualisation can be helpful ways to identify our pelvic floor.
- Once we have identified how to tighten and loosen our pelvic floor we can then hold these positions for longer and longer and perform several repetitions. Aim for 10 repetitions performed several times per day.
- Pelvic floor exercises can be performed when we are lying down, sitting or standing, and so can be done anywhere.

YOUR *Weekly* CHALLENGE . . . .

This week your challenge is to strengthen your core. Perform the suggested activities several times this week. Start with locating your pelvic floor and strengthen this before you move on to general strengthening exercises. If you experience pain consult a physiotherapist to guide you through these exercises.

recognise overtraining

It is quite common for people to become overzealous with their exercise regimen. The endorphins, adrenalin and serotonin released during exercise can be addictive to the point that individuals seek to exercise at all costs rather than listen to their bodies when they need a rest. Now this chapter is not referring to the exerciser who is doing the recommended amount of exercise for health (e.g. walking for 30 minutes most days per week) but is aimed more at individuals who are pushing their bodies to the limit in order to achieve a new level of fitness, a particular health goal, or who is competing in a sporting event.

It is important to recognise when you might be overtraining to avoid the long-term consequences that can come from over-exercising. This of course does not mean that exercise should be limited indefinitely that you should be put off exercising completely, but rather that you need to heed your body's warning signs that a rest day might be needed or when training intensity needs to be reduced for a period of time to allow your body to recover completely. This is particularly important for those whose vocation is sport – such as competitive athletes – but it is equally applicable to the rest of us who participate in sport and exercise as a way to keep physically fit.

Health TIP . . . .

Overtraining and not resting can result in injury and fatigue no matter how fit you are.

Why Is Rest from Training So Important?

Rest days from training are critical for a variety of reasons. Some are physiological and some are psychological. In particular rest from training allows:

- Muscles to repair, rebuild and strengthen
- The body to replenish energy stores and repair damaged tissues
- The body to remove the chemicals that build up as a result of cell activity during exercise, such as lactic acid
- Brain chemicals to replenish that are depleted during exercise, such as dopamine, endorphins and serotonin
- A better balance between home, work and fitness goals to be achieved

If we do not allow our bodies to recover from exercise and training we can develop the symptoms of overtraining.

Alarm Signs That You Are Overtraining

According to Sports Medicine expert, Dr Elizabeth Quinn, signs you may be suffering from overtraining include[1,4]:

- Washed-out feeling, tired, drained, lack of energy
- Mild leg soreness, general aches and pains
- Pain in muscles and joints
- Sudden drop in performance
- Insomnia
- Headaches
- Decreased immunity (increased number of colds and sore throats)
- Decrease in training capacity/intensity
- Moodiness and irritability
- Depression
- Loss of enthusiasm for exercise or sport
- Decreased appetite
- Increased incidence of injuries

How a Diagnosis of Overtraining Is Made

Along with the above signs you may be able to detect overtraining by tracking your heart rate with something called the orthostatic heart rate test.

This test was developed by Heikki Rusko who used it while working with cross country skiers[2].

To obtain this measurement:

- Lie down and rest comfortably for 10 minutes at same time each day (morning is best)
- At the end of 10 minutes, record your heart rate in beats per minute
- Then stand up
- After 15 seconds, take a second heart rate measurement in beats per minute
- After 90 seconds, take a third heart rate measurement in beats per minute
- After 120 seconds, take a fourth heart rate measurement in beats per minute

If you are well rested you will show a consistent heart rate between measurements, but Rusko found a marked increase (10 beats per minute or more) in the 120-second-post-standing measurement of those on the verge of overtraining. Such a change may indicate that you have not recovered from a previous workout, are fatigued or stressed, and it may be helpful to reduce training or rest another day before performing another workout.

A training log that includes a note about how you feel each day can help you notice downward trends and decreased enthusiasm. It is important to listen to your body signals and rest when you feel tired.

You can also ask those around you if they think you are exercising too much. Although a very subjective measure, it is often interesting to hear what those closest to you think about your training frequency.

How You Can Recover From Overtraining

If you suspect you are overtraining, start with the following:

- Rest and recover – reduce or stop exercise and allow yourself a few days of rest.
- Hydrate – drink plenty of fluids.
- Get a sports massage – this may help relax you mentally and physically.
- Begin cross training – by varying your training, different muscle types are working whilst others recover. This also helps to avoid mental fatigue from participating in the same activity all the time.
- Get enough sleep – ensuring consistent, adequate sleep throughout the week has been shown to help safeguard against overtraining syndrome[3].
- Get adequate nutrition – feed your body with the building blocks needed for repair and recover, including adequate protein, good fats and some complex carbohydrates in the form of wholegrains (rather than processed foods).

Keep in mind that severe overtraining may take weeks or even months to recover from.

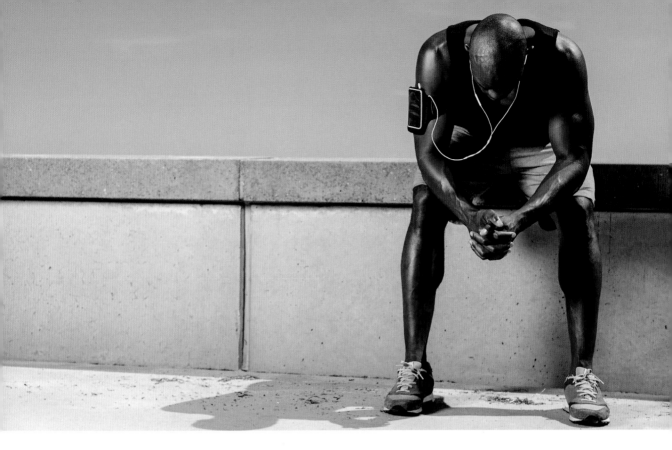

Take Home Points

Overtraining can occur when rest is not adequate between training sessions.

- It leads to fatigue, mental health changes, injuries, reduced physical performance and reduced immunity.
- Rest in between hard exercise training sessions is important to avoid overtraining.
- If you suspect you are suffering from overtraining some strategies to recovering from this include ensuring adequate hydration, nutrition, rest and sleep.
- Asking someone who is close to you if they think you are overtraining might be a helpful, subjective way to assess whether you need to incorporate some rest days into your training schedule.

YOUR *Weekly* CHALLENGE · · · · · · · · · · · · · · · · · · ·

This week your challenge is to avoid overtraining by incorporating rest days into your program. This might involve a complete day off exercise or just reducing the intensity of training on a particular day to some less-intense forms of exercises/stretches.

boost your metabolism

Aside from what you may have heard, your metabolism is not static but dynamic. Meaning that the speed of your metabolism can be changed. Many people feel that they are stuck with a certain type of metabolism; either slow or fast. This is simply not the case. Your metabolism can be sped up or slowed down depending on certain factors that we will discuss in this chapter.

Before we examine the factors that can boost the speed of our metabolism let us explore what exactly we mean by the word 'metabolism' and how we can determine how fast or slow our individual metabolism is at the moment.

What Exactly Is Metabolism?

Metabolism refers to all the chemical processes going on continuously inside our bodies that maintain normal body functioning, including building and repairing our body tissues.

The amount of energy, measured in Calories (Cals) or kilojoules (kJ) that our body burns at any given time is affected by our metabolism. If we eat and drink more Cals/kJ than we can burn via our metabolism or through physical activity we store the extra mainly as body fat. The rate at which our body burns energy is called our metabolic rate.

Health FACT · · · · · · · · · · · · · · · · ·

Our metabolic rate can be calculated by:

Basal Metabolic Rate + Physical Activity + Thermic Effect of Food = Metabolic Rate

How To Calculate Your Metabolic Rate

IF YOU EAT OR DRINK THIS...	YOU NEED TO WALK FOR...	YOU NEED TO JOG FOR...
Soft drink (375 mL)	1 hr 7 mins	19 min
Large juice (650 mL)	2 hrs 8 min	37 min
Chocolate bar (60 g)	2 hrs 15 min	39 min
Flavoured milk (500 mL)	3 hrs 7 min	53 min
Meat pie	3 hrs 5 min	53 min
2 slices pizza	6 hrs 3 min	1 hr 27 min
Fish and chips (battered & fried)	6 hrs 53 min	1 hr 40 min

To calculate your current metabolic rate (or total energy expenditure for the day) you need to take into consideration your resting metabolic rate called your 'basal metabolic rate', the energy you used during planned and incidental physical activity, as well as the Calorie-burning effect of breaking down food (called the 'thermic effect'). These are briefly described below.

Basal metabolic rate (BMR) This is the amount of Cals or kJ burned at rest. BMR includes the energy the body uses to keep all its systems functioning correctly. It accounts for the largest amount of energy expended daily (50-80 per cent of your daily energy use). Our BMR is largely determined by the amount of muscle we have. The more muscle we have, the more energy we will burn at rest. This is why men tend to be able to eat more than women and not gain weight. An average 70 kg man has a BMR of around 7,100 kJ (1690 Cals) per day, while an average 70 kg woman has a BMR of around 5,900 kJ (1404 Cals) per day. The difference is the amount of lean muscle mass the average man would have compared to the average woman.

Energy used during physical activity Physical activity burns energy and contributes to our metabolic rate - in fact it can contribute to as much as 20 per cent of our daily energy use. During heavy physical exertion, the muscles may burn through as much as 3 000 kJ (716 Cals) per hour. Keep in mind that foods that are high in sugar and/or fat content may be very energy dense and therefore you need to do a lot of physical activity to burn these foods off. This is shown in the table above. An apple takes only 10 minutes of exercise to burn off, so it pays to eat as fresh and unprocessed as possible. Staying away from excess processed fats and sugars means we have less to burn off during the day.

Thermic effect of food This is the energy you use to eat, digest and metabolise food. It contributes about 5-10 per cent of your energy use. Interestingly, hot spicy foods can have a significant thermic effect, meaning that they can speed up your metabolism.

So you can see that our metabolic rate is comprised of multiple parts, and to calculate it exactly poses a challenge as it may change from day to day.

An easier way to determine if your metabolism is working adequately is to see what your weight is doing from week to week. If you are eating less and engaging in lots of activity but still not losing weight then this is a sign that your metabolism is being hampered by one or more of the factors listed below.

What Can Affect Your Metabolism?

Your metabolism can be influenced by multiple factors working in combination, including:

- Amount of lean muscle tissue - muscle burns energy rapidly
- Amount of body fat - fat cells are 'sluggish' and burn far less energy than most other tissues and organs of the body
- Crash dieting, starving or fasting - encourages the body to slow the metabolism to conserve energy. Our basal metabolic rate can drop by up to 15 per cent due to dieting or fasting
- Age - metabolism slows with age (as discussed further below)
- Hormonal imbalance - Hormonal imbalances can influence how quickly or slowly the body burns energy. These hormonal imbalances can include thyroid conditions, a progesterone/oestrogen imbalance, as well as insulin resistance. Thyroid conditions are discussed further below
- Infection or illness - our bodies have to work harder to build new tissues and to create an immune response
- Amount of physical activity - hard-working muscles need plenty of energy to burn. Regular exercise increases muscle mass and teaches the body to burn energy at a faster rate, even when at rest
- Drugs - some like caffeine or nicotine, can increase our metabolism (although smoking is not recommended!)
- Dietary deficiencies - for example, a diet low in iodine reduces thyroid function and slows the metabolism

Now that we have looked at what can affect our metabolism let's consider some things we can implement into our lifestyles to speed up our metabolism.

Ways to Naturally Speed Up Your Metabolism

Listed below are some ways to naturally boost our metabolism.

Avoid Meal Skipping Skipping meals convinces our bodies that we are in starvation mode. The result is a slowing of our metabolic rate. Try to eat a small meal or snack every 3-4 hours. This means you will be eating around 5-6 meals per day.

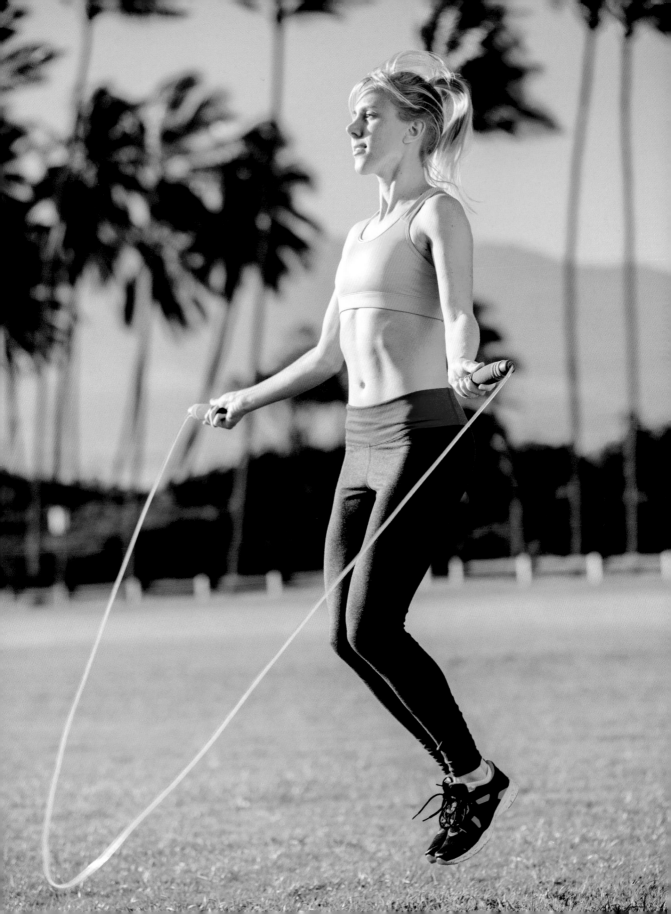

Avoid Dieting Similarly, dieting to the extreme, whereby we reduce our Calorie intake to very low levels, usually lower than 1200 Calories for women and 1400 Calories for men, will cause our metabolism to slow down. Dieting to this extreme can also cause our lean muscle mass to waste away, which further reduces our metabolism.

Be Active Exercise stimulates thyroid hormone secretion and raises our metabolic rate. It is recommended that you do at least 30 minutes per day of some form of exercise to boost your metabolic rate for 1-2 hours after you have finished exercising.

Increase Lean Muscle For every 1 kilogram of muscle that you have, you burn an extra 100 Calories at rest. This means that if you have plenty of lean muscle you will be able to burn a lot more of the food you eat without storing it as body fat. Resistance training in the form of either body weight exercises or fixed/dumbbell style exercises build muscle. Try incorporating some of these types of exercises into your weekly routine to maintain your muscle mass.

Sleep and Rest It is important that we get enough sleep and rest to maintain our metabolism. Those of us who are highly stressed, not sleeping well, or not taking time to wind down will find that our metabolisms will eventually slow as a result.

Eat a Nutrient-Rich Diet A diet rich in vitamin C, selenium, B vitamins, zinc, vitamin E, iodine and L-tyrosine can help to boost your metabolism. Make sure you are eating plenty of fresh fruits, vegetables, fish and lean meat in order to get enough of these essential nutrients from your diet.

Incorporating these simple activities into our daily schedules helps to boost our metabolic rate. However there are two situations that will affect our metabolisms independently of our actions and that is due to normal ageing or to thyroid disease.

Why Does Your Metabolism Slow Down As You Get Older?

People tend to put on fat as they age, partly because the body slowly loses muscle from about the age of 30 years. It is not clear whether muscle loss is a result of the ageing process or because many people are less active as they age. Both are probably factors. In order to maintain as much muscle mass as possible and therefore help to maintain our metabolism as we age, it is important to incorporate some exercise into our daily life. As the saying goes, 'Use it or lose it'.

Could It Be Your Thyroid?

Thyroid hormones secreted from our thyroid gland help regulate our metabolism. This gland is located in the front of our neck just above the collar bones. Thyroid hormones not only regulate our metabolism but also our organ function, heart rate, cholesterol levels, body weight, energy levels, muscle contraction and relaxation, skin and hair texture, bowel function, fertility, menstrual period, memory, mood and other vital processes.

When our thyroid is functioning too slowly we are suffering from a medical condition known as an underactive thyroid. This condition can lead to some significant signs and often presents late to the doctor's surgery because it can come on slowly over a period of months or in some cases years.

Hypothyroidism (underactive thyroid) In this condition the metabolism slows because the thyroid gland does not release enough hormones. Some of the symptoms of hypothyroidism include unusual weight gain, lethargy, intolerance to cold temperatures, depression, hair loss especially the outer third of your eyebrows, fluid retention, dry skin and hair, heavy menstrual period, and constipation. You may have all of these symptoms or just a few.

A common cause is the autoimmune condition Hashimoto's disease. Nutritional deficiencies of iodine, selenium, and L-tyrosine may also cause an underactive thyroid, as will female hormone imbalances (discussed further in *Simple Health Habit #40 Balancing Your Sex Hormones*) and high stress levels. There is some suggestion from studies that excessive consumption of soy-based foods may decrease thyroid hormone in the body, as well as excessive ingesting of fluoride from drinking water.

An underactive thyroid can be diagnosed by a blood test and if your thyroid gland is enlarged or a lump can be felt then a thyroid ultrasound scan may also be requested. Keep in mind with thyroid testing the optimal levels for thyroid stimulating hormone (TSH) are between 0.2 and 2.0. This is often the only test requested by your doctor. I recommend paying for the additional test of reverse T3 as well as a spot urine iodine test.

If your reverse T3 level is higher than 230, it is a sign that your metabolism is being slowed down by stress levels and/or selenium deficiency. In this case a trial of selenium supplement – 200 mcg daily for 3 months – as well as checking your urine iodine levels would be helpful. If you have an iodine deficiency detected on urine iodine testing consider taking an iodine supplement for 3–6 months. I recommend consulting with your health care practitioner before taking any supplements however, including iodine, as excess iodine in the case of Hashimoto's disease can actually make it worse.

Once a diagnosis is made of a thyroid condition the treatment may also involve medication. Medications that may be used to supplement your thyroid function in the case of an underactive thyroid include levothyroxine and thyroid extract. Both can be effective depending on the individual. The benefit of thyroid extract, I find, is that it contains a mixture of all the thyroid hormones and not just one (levothyroxine contains just one of the 4 known thyroid hormones). This often helps in times when individuals do not respond to levothyroxine i.e. they still do not feel any better and cannot lose weight.

If you suspect you have a thyroid condition speak to your doctor about getting some initial testing.

Take Home Points

We are not stuck with a fast or slow metabolism.

- Our metabolism can be sped up or slowed down depending on our lifestyles.
- Our metabolism is determined by the amount of energy we burn at rest, the amount of physical activity we do and the thermic effect of food.
- Factors that will speed up our metabolism include: avoiding dieting, not skipping meals, being active, building our muscle mass, and making sure we are getting enough sleep and rest.
- As we age our metabolism will naturally slow down, mostly due to a decline in our muscle mass from being inactive.
- It is important that we keep up our activity levels as we age to maintain our muscle tissue. This is because muscle is very metabolically active and will boost our resting metabolisms.
- Thyroid disease is also a relatively common cause of slowed metabolism. It is caused by autoimmune conditions but also may be caused by stress, hormone imbalances, and nutrient deficiencies in our diet.
- Diagnosis of thyroid conditions involves bloods testing, urine iodine testing, and in some cases a thyroid ultrasound scan.
- Thyroid conditions can be easily diagnosed and relatively easily treated using a combination of natural supplements, depending on whether a deficiency exists, as well as medication if needed.

YOUR *Weekly* CHALLENGE . . . .

This week your challenge is to choose 2 things to work on to boost your metabolism. They could be dietary or exercise-based. If you suspect you might have a thyroid condition consider having some testing undertaken by your doctor.

boost your immunity

Our immune system acts as our defence against invading germs. It is comprised of a complex set of tissues, cells and molecules which specialise in defending against infections. When our immune system is functioning optimally infections are kept at bay. There is, however, a degree of variance between people and the efficiency of their immune systems. This can be due to genetic differences in immune function but also due to some environmental factors.

Health FACT ·

The average adult has 2-3 upper respiratory tract infections per year whist the average child has 6-10 per year[1].

What Affects Your Immunity?

Multiple environmental factors impact on our immune system function but, by and large, the most common factors include[2]:

- Chronic stress
- Depression
- Lack of sunshine (vitamin D)
- Lack of sleep
- Poor diet
- Lack of vitamin A, C, E, B6, B12 and folate
- Lack of zinc, iron and copper

- Certain medications such as corticosteroids and chemotherapy
- Smoking
- Long-term pollution exposure
- Poor hygiene

These factors not only account for differences in individual immunity but may also account for why we may be healthy one year and then recurrently sick with infections the following year. It is not uncommon for me to encounter this in clinical practice. A patient who, for example, has been emotionally stressed for a prolonged period of time may find that they are unable to shake a cold or flu virus where they have previously had a very resilient immune system. Once the stressful situation passes and life returns to normal the person's immune function seems to be restored to previous levels.

Top Immune Boosters

The following strategies have been proven to be beneficial in boosting our immunity:

- **Reduce Stress Levels** High stress hormone levels can impair immunity and make us susceptible to recurrent infections. Consider taking a holiday and resting if you find that you are recurrently sick.

- **Try Hypnosis** There is some evidence to suggest that this may be beneficial in improving immunity in cases of viral illnesses including herpes and the common cold[1].

- **Get Enough Sunshine (& Vitamin D)** Studies suggest that vitamin D deficiency may precipitate the development of autoimmune diseases[1]. Autoimmune diseases are those in which the immune system starts to attack our own bodies and includes diseases such as multiple sclerosis, rheumatoid arthritis, inflammatory bowel disease, and type 1 diabetes. There is no established cause for autoimmune diseases but one growing area of research suggests that adequate vitamin D levels may help to prevent these diseases from developing[1].

- **Sleep Well** Poor sleep quality and not getting enough sleep has been linked to increased susceptibility to the common cold. It is important to get a good night's sleep to protect immune system function[3].

- **Move** Studies confirm that exercise helps to boost our immune system function.

- **Deep Breathe** There is some research to suggest that deep breathing techniques help to boost immune system function[1].

- **Eat Immune Boosting Foods** Eating plenty of fresh fruits and vegetables, nuts, seeds and fish helps to boost our immune systems; as does moderate amounts of cocoa/dark chocolate, green tea, oysters and shiitake mushrooms[1].

- **Add Some Spice** The spices turmeric and paprika may help to improve immune system function as does garlic and ginger[1]. Try adding these into your cooking.

- **Boost Omega 3** Omega 3 fish oil has been shown to boost immune function by activating B-cells[3], which is a key component in forming long-term immunity. Consider supplementing your family's diet with a good quality omega 3 fish oil, especially if your family does not regularly consume omega 3-rich fish like salmon, tuna, herring, sardines or mackerel.

- **Take Probiotics** A large percentage of our immune response is in our gut and this immune response depends on the presence of beneficial bacteria that live in our gut; namely the lactobacillus and bifidobacterium species. If there is an imbalance of bacteria living in our gut due to lifestyle, stress, medication use or other factors then we may become more susceptible to infections[1]. Try taking a good-quality probiotic daily if you are experiencing recurrent infections. There is some current thinking that fermented foods such as kefir, sauerkraut and kimchi might be a more bioavailable way to introduce probiotics into our intestinal tracts. These can be inexpensively made at home and a small amount eaten regularly.

- **Increase Vitamin C** This is a key nutrient to improve immunity[3]. Many fruits and vegetables do not contain the required daily amounts due to food processing practices. Consider taking up to 1000 mg a day in the winter months.

- **Increase Zinc** Likewise, zinc is also a key ingredient required for immune function[3]. Zinc is found in animal products, beans, nuts and certain types of seafood. In winter months consider taking a zinc supplement of around 25-30 mg a day.

- **Reduce Sugar** Sugar intake can inhibit immune function[3]. Consider limiting the amount of hidden, processed sugar you consume such as that found in breakfast cereals, muesli bars, biscuits and lollies.

- **Consider Herbal Medicine** If you find that you just cannot seem to shake an infection you can try herbal medicines containing Astragalus and/or Echinacea[1]. Astragalus is commonly used in Chinese medicine and has been shown in several studies to help modulate immune function[3]. Echinacea has been shown to be helpful in the early treatment of the common cold, reducing its severity and duration[3]. Also, specifically for urinary tract infections, concentrated cranberry extract may be helpful[1]. Avoid drinking cranberry juice – rather take it in capsule form as sugar is often added to sweeten the juice product. Other herbs such as olive leaf extract, mushroom extract and green tea extract are yet to be properly evaluated in research but may have a positive effect. Always choose good quality, pure products due to the effects of unknown additives in poorer quality products.

Consider, too, speaking with your health-care practitioner if you are experiencing recurrent infections as this may be a sign of a specific medical condition requiring more specialised diagnosis and treatment. More than a few infections per year, especially if they are severe or take more than a few weeks to completely clear, need to be looked into further. Infections that suggest a compromised immune system include recurrent mouth ulcers and cold sores, genital herpes, as well as shingles. These all warrant further investigation to ensure there are no underlying health concerns.

Take Home Points

Our immune systems protect us from outside germs and infections.

- When our immune system functions well we are able to quickly fight infections.
- If our immune system is working efficiently we will not even realise we are fighting an infection. All we may feel is a little fatigued or have mild body aches.
- If, however, our immune system is compromised we are unable to fight infections quickly and find that we become susceptible to recurrent illnesses.
- Our immune system can be compromised by a number of lifestyle factors, including poor nutrition, stress, poor sleep, as well as environmental factors.
- In order to boost our immune system and safeguard our bodies from developing infections we can trial strategies such as getting enough sleep and rest, reducing our stress levels, reducing sugar in our diets and making sure we are eating enough fruits and vegetables as well as fish.
- Supplements that may help to boost our immunity include omega 3 fish oil, probiotics, zinc, vitamin C, Astragalus and Echinacea. Others that may be helpful but as yet are unproven in scientific studies include olive leaf extract, green tea extract and mushroom compounds.
- Recurrent infections, especially infections indicating significant immune compromise such as cold sores, genital herpes, mouth ulcers and shingles, should be investigated by your health-care practitioner to ensure there is no underlying cause.

YOUR *Weekly* CHALLENGE . . . .

This week your challenge is to take at least 2 measures to boost your immune system function, such as eating more fish and taking a vitamin D supplement. If you are suffering from recurrent infections consider speaking with your health-care practitioner to diagnose the underlying cause.

balance your sex hormones

Our sex hormones play such an important part in our overall health and well-being. Essentially they make us who we are. Studies have shown that not only do sex hormones determine whether we develop male or female characteristics but they also influence our brain to the point of directing whether we think like a man or a woman. When we are imbalanced in our sex hormone levels there can be significant detrimental consequences to our physical, mental and sexual health. I have been surprised to find that so many of my patients have sex hormone problems and it seems these problems are starting at a much younger age. In times gone by, sex hormone imbalances just kicked in as we got older (for example, menopause). But hormone problems are now being influenced by modern-day living and presenting much earlier; not surprisingly the biggest of these influences being stress and an unhealthy lifestyle.

So how do we know if we have a sex hormone imbalance and what can we do about it? Before I answer this let us explore the role of the different sex hormones in the body; namely oestrogen, progesterone and testosterone.

Health FACT . . . .

Hormone imbalances can start at any age from puberty and can significantly impact your physical and emotional health. Luckily, natural solutions to rebalance your hormones can be very effective.

Your Sexy Hormones

Sex hormones are important for both men and women to maintain sexual and reproductive function. Women need appropriate amounts of oestrogen and progesterone and a small amount of testosterone; whilst men need mainly testosterone and a small amount of oestrogen. When hormones are balanced they serve these important functions in men and women:

	ROLES IN WOMEN	ROLES IN MEN
Oestrogen	• Produced mainly by the ovaries • Small amount produced from body fat stores and from adrenal glands • Causes egg to mature, ready for ovulation • Thickens the lining of the womb • Maintains vaginal lubrication • Helps to build bone • Helps to protect the heart • Assists in the control of fluid and electrolyte balance within the body, ensuring that skin retains moisture	• Produced from body fat stores • Regulates testosterone function • Helps with sperm development
Progesterone	• Produced in the ovary after ovulation by a structure known as corpus luteum • Maintains lining of womb ready for implantation of embryo • Maintains stable mood • Helps with sleep	• As yet unknown role in men
Testosterone	• Produced mainly by the ovaries and adrenal glands and a small amount in body fat • Maintains libido • Could have a role in cognition and memory	• Produced by the testes • Sperm development • Facial hair growth • Voice deepening • Muscle and bone growth • Maintains libido • Amplifies motivation, competitiveness and confidence

When there is an imbalance of our hormone levels a range of symptoms can occur as the table on the opposite page outlines (adapted from *The Hormone Diet*[1]).

As this shows, our hormones lie in a delicate balance; when we have too much we can develop symptoms and when we do not have enough we also develop symptoms. So what are the main culprits leading to an imbalance of hormone levels?

	EXCESS	LOW
Oestrogen	• Spider or varicose veins • Cellulite • Heavy menstrual bleeding • Breast disease • Prostate enlargement • Erectile dysfunction • Breast growth (men) • Irritability, mood swings, anxiety • Headaches/migraines (especially before menstrual periods in women) • Abdominal fat gain 'love handles' (men) • Fat gain around hips (women)	• Dry or sagging skin • Hair loss • Dry eyes (women) • Thinning skin • Mood swings or depression • Infertility • No menstrual period • Painful intercourse • Urinary incontinence • Fatigue • Hot flushes • Headaches or migraines • Poor memory or concentration • Irritability • Loss of libido • Loss of bone density such as osteoporosis • Sleep problems
Progesterone	• Acne • Depression • Water retention • Weight gain or difficulty losing weight	• Dry skin • Spider or varicose veins • Hair loss • Short menstrual cycle (<28 days) or excessively long bleeding times (>6 days) • PMS characterised by breast soreness, anxiety, sleep problems, headaches, menstrual spotting, water retention and bloating • Infertility or absent menstrual periods • Breast disease • Water retention • Irritability • Anxiety • Loss of libido • Headaches or migraines • Difficulty falling or staying asleep
Testosterone	• Acne • Abnormal facial or body hair growth (women) • Hair loss on scalp • Infertility • Prostate enlargement • Dark underarm pigmentation (women) • Irritability, aggression • Fat gain around abdomen (women) • Sugar or carbohydrate cravings (women) • Fatty liver (women)	• Dry skin • Thinning skin • Painful intercourse • Heart disease (men) • Low sex drive • Depression or anxiety • Poor memory or concentration • Erectile dysfunction • Loss of morning erections • Fatigue • Poor exercise tolerance • Loss of muscle tone • Fat gain around abdomen 'love handles' (men and women) • Headaches or migraines (men) • Loss of motivation or competitive edge • Loss of bone density or osteoporosis (men)

Your Hormone Assailants

A number of factors from lifestyle to genetic to even normal ageing can result in hormone imbalances. The following, however, are some of the most common culprits to disrupting hormone balance that I encounter in clinical practice for both men and women.

Stress The higher the stress levels the lower the progesterone levels in women and the lower the testosterone levels in men, as the body essentially 'steals' these hormones to increase production of the stress hormone cortisol.

Alcohol Consistent heavy alcohol consumption can impair testosterone levels in men due to a direct toxic effect on the testes. In women it can impair oestrogen and progesterone levels causing menstrual period problems, infertility and even miscarriage.

Caffeine Caffeine increases stress hormone release which can, in turn, lower progesterone production in women and testosterone production in men.

Diet A diet that is high in sugary, refined foods stimulates excessive insulin release. High insulin levels can disrupt oestrogen production and inhibit progesterone release.

Abdominal fat stores Carrying too much body fat around the middle can raise oestrogen levels causing an oestrogen-to-progesterone imbalance.

Lack of exercise Exercise helps to boost testosterone levels as well as reduce stress hormone levels. A lack of exercise has been associated with lower circulating levels of testosterone.

Lack of sleep Sleep deprivation causes excess stress hormone release, which, as mentioned above, can disrupt hormone balance.

Ageing As we age our production of hormones naturally declines. At menopause, hormone levels drastically reduce, which can cause various symptoms including hot flushes, poor sleep and memory, irritability, low sex drive, vaginal dryness, and a change in body fat stores to be more centred around the abdomen. Andropause is a term used to describe the male version of menopause when testosterone levels decline. This happens from about the age of 40 for men and results in a lowering of sex drive, muscle mass, and an increase in body fat stores. There are various complementary and hormonal treatments available for the management of these symptoms.

Environmental hormone disruptors There is preliminary research to suggest that the chemicals and hormones in our food, cosmetics, plastics and cleaning products may disrupt our hormones. As much as possible choose hormone-free meat and chicken products. Also choose natural cosmetics free from preservatives such as parabens. With regards to plastics make sure they as BPA-free e.g. drink bottles, containers.

A Word on Improving Your Sex Drive

Many factors can influence sex drive including low testosterone levels, fatigue, pain, anxiety and stress, depression, relationship stress and poor communication, as well erectile dysfunction. In order to improve your sex drive you need to look at the factors affecting your libido and address these specifically.

If low testosterone is the issue (confirmed on pathology testing) then a trial of the following may be warranted:

- **Tribulus terrestris** - may be helpful in improving testosterone levels in men and women. It is best taken on an empty stomach at a dose of 500-1000 mg per day.
- **Indol-3-Carbinol (I3C)** - this is an extract from cruciferous vegetables and may help boost testosterone levels by preventing its conversion to oestrogen. Take 200 mg twice daily.
- **Testosterone** - this is used in cases where testosterone levels are confirmed as very low, usually in men over the age of 60 years and postmenopausal women who are experiencing very low libido due to testosterone deficiency. This is prescribed by your health practitioner.

How to Balance Your Hormones Naturally

If you can relate to any of the symptoms of hormone imbalance mentioned here, then consider the following suggestions to naturally balance your hormone levels.

FOR WOMEN & MEN

Firstly work on reducing stress levels, get enough sleep and exercise, watch the amount of coffee, alcohol and sugar you consume, and look to improve your personal relationships. These general lifestyle factors will all help to rebalance hormone levels. Specifically, there are some supplements as well as hormone medications that may be needed in certain situations. It is best that you consult with your health practitioner before taking these as they may interact with other supplements or medications that you are taking, or may have side-effects that you need to be aware of.

FOR PRE-MENOPAUSAL WOMEN

Supplements that may be helpful in restoring hormone balance if you have not yet reached menopause include:

- **Chasteberry (Vitex)** This increases the progesterone levels and is usually best taken on an empty stomach at a dose of 200 mg per day for 1 to 6 months at a time.
- **Indol-3-Carbinol** This is an active ingredient extracted from broccoli and other cruciferous vegetables. It is known to increase the breakdown and excretion of excess oestrogen. Take 200 mg twice daily for 1-3 months.

- **Evening primrose oil** This may help improve progesterone levels and reduce symptoms of painful periods and breast pain prior to menstruation. Take 1000-2000 mg per day with food.
- **Milk Thistle (St Mary's Thistle or Silymarin)** This extract has been shown to help support liver detoxification and therefore improve oestrogen metabolism. Take 140 mg of silymarin 3 times daily with or without food.
- **Omega-3 fatty acids** Taking a good quality fish oil supplement may help to relieve the symptoms of painful periods. You could also try increasing your intake of omega-3 rich foods such as linseed (flaxseed) or oily fish such as salmon, sardines and mackerel.
- **Vitamin B6** this may help with PMS symptoms and irritability. Take 50-100 mg daily.
- **5-hydroxytryptophan (5-HTP)** This is used in the body to synthesise the happy hormone serotonin, and may be helpful in alleviating PMS and mood swings. Take 100 mg daily on an empty stomach.
- **Progesterone cream** This is made by compounding pharmacies and can be used if you have a low progesterone level and significant symptoms as a result. Usually it is given from days 14-28 of your menstrual cycle and applied either to the skin or into the vagina. It must be prescribed by your health practitioner.

SPECIFIC CONDITIONS – ENDOMETRIOSIS, FIBROIDS, POLYCYSTIC OVARY SYNDROME (PCOS) PRE-MENSTRUAL SYNDROME (PMS)

These conditions are usually a sign of hormone imbalance and, as such, all of the lifestyle suggestions as well as one or more of the above supplements may be of help. In some cases the use of the oral contraceptive pill may be warranted. Once again it is worth discussing this further with your health-care practitioner.

FOR MENOPAUSAL WOMEN

Menopause is not a disease as some would like to suggest but rather part of the inevitable natural progression of women's bodies. If you have no symptoms then there is no need to treat with hormones or natural medications. If, however, your life is being significantly impacted by the hormone imbalances that can come with menopause then it is worth speaking with your health-care practitioner about the following options for management:

- **Black Cohosh** Acts like oestrogen in the body and is used to treat hot flushes, night sweats, vaginal dryness and urinary urgency. It is usually taken as a 40 mg dose twice daily on an empty stomach. It is not advisable to take any compounds that act like oestrogen in the body if you have had a history of breast cancer or endometrial cancer.

- **Red Clover** Contains high quantities of plant-based oestrogens that may improve menopausal symptoms. You could trial taking 80 mg per day.

- **St John's Wort** This acts as a mild serotonin booster and may help to alleviate the symptoms of hot flushes and mood swings.

- **Medications** Sometimes medications are needed in the treatment of menopausal symptoms. These can include clonidine for hot flushes, low-dose anti-depressants or hormonal treatments, which are discussed further below.

- **Hormone Treatment** Sometimes the use of hormone treatment is needed to relieve menopausal symptoms of hot flushes, irritability, poor sleep and low sex drive. The goal with hormone treatment is to take the lowest effective dose that controls your symptoms and not to stay on it for many years once symptoms are controlled (generally less than 5 years). Hormone therapy can come with risks and so it is worth speaking with your health-care practitioner about this option and then weighing up the pros and cons for your situation.

Keep in mind, too, with menopause that it is important to maintain healthy bone mass by getting enough exercise as well as calcium and vitamin D intake.

FOR MEN

The key to maintaining male hormone health is to maintain healthy testosterone levels. Thus, the measures described above for improving sex drive are also applicable to male health. A note to add regarding exercise – short sharp bursts of exercise in the form of interval training may be more beneficial to men needing to boost testosterone levels rather than endurance type training, which can lower testosterone levels long-term.

SPECIFIC CONDITIONS – ENLARGED PROSTATE, ERECTILE DYSFUNCTION AND PROSTATE CANCER

These conditions all have specific treatments that are worth discussing with your health-care practitioner if you are experiencing any concerning symptoms. There are, however, some lifestyle factors that have been shown to be effective, including maintaining a healthy body weight, a diet rich in vegetables, fruit, fish and low in red meat. These have all been shown to be effective in promoting men's health. Additionally, in the case of enlarged prostate, the saw palmetto plant taken as a supplement (containing 320 mg per day) may be helpful.

Take Home Points

Our sex hormones lie in a delicate balance.

When they are in balance we have normal sexual and reproductive function and generally feel well.

- If our sex hormones become imbalanced we can experience a range of symptoms from low sex drive, menstrual problems, weight gain, fluid retention, headaches, mood swings, low motivation and even depression.

- There are many causes for disrupted hormones but the common ones are related to high stress levels, too much sugary foods in the diet, carrying too much abdominal fat, drinking too much coffee and alcohol, as well as not getting enough sleep or exercise.

- Hormones decline as we age, but there are natural ways to boost hormone levels as well as taking hormone treatment, if needed, to keep symptoms at bay.

- Beneficial natural supplements for pre-menopausal women include chasteberry (vitex), indol-3-carbinol, silymarin, vitamin B6, evening primrose oil, omega-3 fatty acids and 5-hydroxytryptophan.

- Beneficial natural supplements for menopausal women may include black cohosh, red clover and St John's Wort.

- Beneficial natural supplements for men may include tribulus and saw palmetto.

- The key to maintaining hormonal health is to maintain a healthy lifestyle, reduce stress levels and maintain positive interpersonal relationships.

YOUR *Weekly* CHALLENGE . . . .

This week your challenge is to identify if you have symptoms of sex hormone imbalance and if so to work on one lifestyle factor listed in this chapter.

simple health habit #41

boost your
happy hormones

We all have happy hormones in our brain and at certain times in our lives and under certain circumstances these can be higher or lower in amount depending on the situation. When our happy hormones become greatly depleted we can develop depression and/or anxiety. This can follow, for example, an extremely stressful period in our lives when we have experienced trauma, or it can just sneak up on us as a result of fatigue and burn-out.

Health FACT

Mental illness is very common. One in 5 Australians aged 16-85 experience mental illness in any year[1]. The most common mental illnesses are anxiety and depression.

I frequently encounter patients who do not realise why they feel so down, have no energy, and cannot sleep. Their happy hormone levels have plummeted so low that they are suffering from the early stages of depression and had no idea that this was happening. One particular patient of mine, a mum of three daughters, came to see me after one of her daughters had in the last 12 months been diagnosed with a serious medical condition. Up to this point she had always been the strong figurehead in the family and kept all the practicalities of home life running. She maintained a brave face and positive attitude until she reached breaking point. She came to see me and told me that she no longer had the motivation to feel happy, felt so guilty for not being able to be present emotionally for her family, and felt exhausted all the time. She was having thoughts of not wanting to wake up in the morning but knew she had to keep going for her daughters. When I suggested that she was suffering from clinical depression she was surprised – the idea had never crossed her mind. Within a few months of starting some treatment, which in her case involved medication as well as counselling, her depression lifted and she was back to being able to cope with the situation at hand.

This example highlights how important it is to have enough happy hormones circulating in our brains to prevent anxiety and depression. With up to 1 in 5 of us developing anxiety and/or depression at some stage in our lives[1] it is paramount that we understand what can affect the levels of happy hormones in our brain so we can hopefully safeguard ourselves from these mental health conditions.

Hidden Suffering

Many people today live their lives under the dark shadow of depression or anxiety and don't realise that they have these mental health conditions. That is because the symptoms can range from mild to severe and so less obvious cases can go undiagnosed. Eventually, though, if depression or anxiety is not treated or well-managed, relationships, careers and overall well-being are significantly impacted. This is often the time when people will seek help, however the recovery is often long and involved.

Another patient of mine, Bill, had been suffering from mild depression for many years without realising. This came about following several rounds of unsuccessful IVF treatment with his then wife. The disappointment of not being able to have children followed by pressures from work caused him to drink wine to cope. After several years of burying his emotions and self-medicating with alcohol he noticed that he no longer had a social life, a fulfilling marriage or a rewarding career. Without realising, Bill had sunk deep into the depths of depression and was on the way to a nervous breakdown. Luckily he sought help with the encouragement of a close friend. That is when Bill came to see me several years ago and we began the journey towards recovery. Although his treatment was sometimes difficult and involved letting go of old thought patterns, old habits and adopting a new way of thinking and living, he is now living a much happier life.

Bill's story is not uncommon and reflects how easy it is in our busy lives to overlook our mental health and well-being. So what exactly are the symptoms of depression or anxiety?

How Do You Know If You Have Clinical Depression?

Symptoms can range from mild to severe but when they significantly impair your quality of life and relationships then doctors refer to that state as 'clinical depression'. To make the diagnosis of clinical depression your doctor will follow the classic textbook definition.

It states that you need to have had at least 5 of the following symptoms present during the same 2-week period[2].

- Depressed mood most of the day, nearly every day, e.g. feeling sad or empty, or often tearful.
- Decreased interest or pleasure in all, or almost all, activities most of the day, nearly every day.
- Significant weight loss when not dieting, or weight gain (e.g. a change of more than 5 per cent of body weight in a month), or decrease or increase in appetite nearly every day.
- Insomnia or increased sleeping nearly every day.
- Agitation or slowed movements.
- Fatigue or loss of energy nearly every day.
- Feelings of worthlessness or excessive or inappropriate guilt nearly every day.
- Diminished ability to think or concentrate, or indecisiveness, nearly every day.
- Recurrent thoughts of death, recurrent suicidal ideation without a specific plan, or a suicide attempt or a specific plan for committing suicide.

Although the above describes a definite diagnosis of depression it is also common to see individuals suffering from lower states of mood without meeting the criteria for severe depression. If you are feeling low for a consistent period of time with or without thoughts of ending your life, then you may be going through a milder case of depression. Seek professional help before it becomes severe.

How Do You Know If You Have Anxiety?

Anxiety is very common and is part of the normal range of human emotions. It can range from mild, low-level anxiousness about certain situations, which may be appropriate given the situation, or it may be excessive. When anxiety begins to rule your happiness, however, and you start to avoid certain situations, this is known as an anxiety disorder.

There are several types of anxiety disorders, including panic disorder, social anxiety disorder, specific phobias and generalised anxiety disorder.

Panic disorder People with this condition experience feelings of terror that strike suddenly and repeatedly with no warning, which is commonly known as a panic attack. Other symptoms of a panic attack include sweating, chest pain, palpitations (unusually strong or irregular heartbeats), and a feeling of choking, which may make the person feel like he or she is having a heart attack or 'going crazy'.

Social anxiety disorder This is also called social phobia. It involves overwhelming worry and self-consciousness about everyday social situations. The worry often centres on a fear of being judged by others, or behaving in a way that might cause embarrassment or lead to ridicule.

Specific phobias A specific phobia is an intense fear of a specific object or situation, such as snakes, heights or flying. The level of fear is usually inappropriate to the situation and may cause the person to avoid common, everyday situations.

Generalized anxiety disorder This disorder involves excessive, unrealistic worry and tension, even if there is little or nothing to provoke the anxiety.

As part of the above anxiety disorders the overall general symptoms of anxiety include[3]:

- Feelings of panic, fear and uneasiness
- Problems sleeping
- Cold or sweaty hands and/or feet
- Shortness of breath
- Heart palpitations
- An inability to be still and calm
- Dry mouth
- Numbness or tingling in the hands or feet
- Nausea
- Muscle tension
- Dizziness

It is quite common to see patients who are unaware that they are suffering specifically from anxiety but have a number of the symptoms above. They often present wanting help with not being able to fall asleep, or waking in the middle of the night and not being able to go back to sleep. This is often the first sign that anxiety is starting to affect your mental well-being. One particular patient of mine, a young woman in her 20s, had a very stressful job with high-level responsibilities for her age. Prior to starting this job she had no problems with sleep, but soon after being promoted to her new role she began finding it difficult to fall asleep at night. She started to panic about not being able to sleep, which perpetuated the problem. She then started having episodes of difficulty breathing, tingling around the mouth and fingertips, feeling lightheaded and faint, and experiencing racing heartbeats. She thought she was having heart troubles and had presented to the emergency department on several occasions only to be sent home with a clean bill of health. When she came to see me she was in quite a state of panic. She spoke quickly, looked exhausted, and found it hard to sit still. We investigated a number of things to rule out any organic cause for her symptoms. When these came back negative, I explained that I thought she was suffering from anxiety related to stress. She was reluctant to accept the diagnosis. When I explained that suffering anxiety did not mean that she was not able to mentally cope with her work situation that she had caused this condition but rather her body was giving her clues that it was time to rest, she was more accepting. We then started the process of unwinding the anxiety response and putting some stress-management strategies in place.

First let us look at what causes depression and anxiety.

What Causes Depression & Anxiety?

There are several theories as to the cause of depression and anxiety, which centre on changes in brain biochemistry. Most focus on 'happy hormone' levels in the brain and how they affect the development and/or perpetuation of anxiety and depression; namely serotonin, dopamine, and gamma-aminobutyric acid (GABA). So what causes changes in these brain biochemistry levels? Some of the potential contributors include:

LONG-TERM STRESS

It is thought that long-term stress alters the nerve pathways in the brain and lowers brain serotonin levels[4]. This may come in the form of a specific traumatic event that is yet to be resolved or ongoing cumulative stresses in your life.

TOO MUCH CAFFEINE

Caffeine is a stimulant and is known to worsen anxiety symptoms[5]. Reducing caffeine to no more than 1-2 cups of coffee or 3-4 cups of tea a day may help to reduce anxiety.

LACK OF SUNLIGHT

Some people are greatly affected by the seasons. Seasonal Affective Disorder (SAD) is a recognised medical condition whereby individuals suffer lowered mood when they are not exposed to enough sunlight for prolonged periods.

PERSONALITY

Some people may be more at risk of depression because of their personality, particularly if they have a tendency to worry a lot, have low self-esteem, are perfectionists, are pessimistic or are sensitive to criticism. Although personality cannot be clinically 'tested' as such, there is a blood test known as whole blood histamine that can examine personality tendencies towards depression and/or anxiety. The lower the number the more likely someone is to be susceptible to anxiety, and the higher the number the more likely someone will be susceptible to depression.

POOR SLEEP

Sleep is needed for restoration of the body. Lack of sleep can lead to depression and anxiety symptoms. Sometimes it can be a vicious cycle as the less sleep you get the more anxious and/or depressed you become, and the more anxious or depressed you become the less sleep you get.

ALCOHOL & DRUG USE

Drug and alcohol use can lead to and result from depression. Many people with depression also have drug and alcohol problems. Over 500 000 Australians will experience depression and a substance-use disorder at the same time at some point in their lives[6].

FAMILY HISTORY

We know there is a genetic link to the susceptibility to depression and anxiety[6]. How strong this link is depends on the number of family members affected, but also depends on internal and external factors independent of family history. So just because a family member has depression or anxiety does not automatically predispose another family member to the same.

How Is Anxiety & Depression Diagnosed?

When making the diagnosis of anxiety and/or depression as a clinician I will also rule out other diseases that may be causing the symptoms. Although rare, these diseases may be 'organic' causes of anxiety and/or depression as opposed to purely biochemical and include, for example, thyroid disease, adrenal gland disorders, Parkinson's disease, dementia or other brain disorders. Usually these conditions will have other symptoms associated with them, which will be evident on further history taking. The testing for these conditions usually involves a blood test, occasionally a brain scan, or other rarely conducted investigations. Your general practitioner is the best person to guide this process.

How Is Anxiety & Depression Treated?

The treatment of anxiety and depression involves a multifactorial approach, meaning that it involves different strategies for different people, and several strategies at the same time for one person.

Practical Strategies One practical approach to reducing anxiety and/or depression symptoms is to stay connected with others. Social isolation will worsen your condition. Try and step out of your comfort zone and stay involved with friends and family even if this means being around them for short periods of time regularly.

Another practical strategy is getting some regular exercise, which has been shown to boost happy hormone levels[7]. I have heard it said by a renowned psychologist and colleague that exercising at sunrise or sunset has the added benefit of boosting even more happy hormones due to the pleasure-inducing experience of gazing on the rising or setting sun.

Trying to eat as healthily as possible eliminates the unwanted effect of poor-quality foods on your mood, including the mood swings that can come from eating sugary foods. Reducing caffeine has also been shown to be beneficial in reducing anxiety levels.

There are some foods that may help to boost happy hormone levels in the brain including walnuts, bananas, oats, chocolate and turkey. This effect would be small but, nevertheless, adding these foods to your diet, of course in moderation, could have some positive effects.

Natural Medications These include the naturally serotonin-boosting herb St John's Wort, as well as the compounds 5-hydroxytryptophan (5-HTP) and S-adenosyl methionine (SAMe). These have been shown to have positive benefits for mild depression and/or anxiety symptoms. Because they can interact with your other medications, including the oral contraceptive pill, make sure you check with your health practitioner before taking them. Additionally, taking a supplement containing gamma-aminobutyric acid (GABA) may be helpful for mild anxiety symptoms. Other natural medications that may be helpful for mild depression and/or anxiety include vitamin B6, vitamin B12, niacin and magnesium.

Pharmaceutical Medications These include the selective serotonin re-uptake inhibitors (SSRIs) and selective noradrenaline re-uptake inhibitors (SNRIs). Examples of these medications include venlafaxine, fluoxetine and sertraline. These medications have been shown to be helpful in cases of moderate to severe depression and it may be necessary to treat for many months to several years to establish steady and happy hormone levels.

Psychological Approaches By far one of the most effective strategies to combating anxiety and/or depression is to have some counselling or behavioural therapy. Often just by having an unbiased, independent health practitioner look at your situation from a different angle and suggest some problem-solving strategies is helpful. Cognitive behavioural therapy in particular has been shown to be very helpful for anxiety symptoms. Interestingly, for mild to moderate depression, psychological counselling has been shown to be more effective than an anti-depressant medication. Often both strategies are used at the same time for the most benefit.

Other psychological approaches that have been shown to be helpful include meditation and mindfulness training, as well as deep breathing. Like any other skill these need to be learnt and practised for maximal results. That said, practising this skill-set does not require hours per day; results can be achieved by practising for only a few minutes per day.

Take Home Points

Anxiety and depression is a common problem that is often overlooked due to the stigma associated with these conditions and their insidious nature.

- They can happen to anyone.
- Anxiety and depression can significantly impact someone's quality of life and relationships and should be considered a real medical problem with effective treatment strategies.
- The symptoms of depression include low mood, lack of interest in activities, loss or increase in appetite, increase or decrease in sleep, lack of interest in sex, and thoughts of hopelessness, worthlessness, guilt and/or death. You may have some of these symptoms or all of them, and they may range from mild to overwhelming in nature and severity.
- The symptoms of anxiety include constant or frequent worrying, feelings of panic or fear, being unable to relax and/or sit still, difficulty sleeping, difficulty concentrating, dry mouth, breathlessness and/or shakiness. Once again these symptoms can range from mild to severe and may be manageable or debilitating.
- A doctor will often undertake several investigations to rule out any organic cause for your anxiety and/or depression before making a final diagnosis.
- The treatment of anxiety and/or depression often involves multiple approaches for the same person and different approaches for different people. These approaches may be practical, such as establishing a regular exercise routine and eating foods rich in nutrition as opposed to empty Calories, or may involve natural medications, pharmaceutical medications and/or counselling. All of these strategies are helpful and your general practitioner is the best person to guide this treatment plan and process.

YOUR *Weekly* CHALLENGE . . . .

This week your challenge is to recognise if you are suffering from anxiety and/or depression. If you feel that you might be and your symptoms are mild you can trial some of the practical strategies listed above. If you feel your symptoms are more severe, then make an appointment with your general practitioner this week to discuss some effective treatment options. You do not need to be living with anxiety or depression.

boost brain alpha waves

Brain alpha waves are a type of brain frequency that signals that your brain is in a wakeful state of resting. This means that you are at peace whilst not being asleep, which involves a different pattern of brain waves. Many of us never reach a place where we activate brain alpha waves due to our busy and stressful lifestyles. Studies have indicated that in order to activate brain alpha waves we need to be doing an activity that we find both enjoyable and calming[1]. This allows brain activity to settle from a chaotic brain-wave pattern into a more harmonious and synchronous brain alpha wave state.

One of the best activities we can do to activate brain alpha waves is mindfulness meditation. The health benefits of mindfulness meditation are extensive and can arguably be attributed to reaching a brain alpha wave state. These benefits include reduced rates of depression and anxiety, lowered blood pressure, increased ability to deal with stress, improved sleep, reduced addictions and cravings, improved memory and concentration, and overall improved mental and physical performance[2,3].

What Is Mindfulness Meditation?

Mindfulness meditation combines two concepts – the art of being mindful and that of meditation. Mindfulness involves paying attention each moment to things as they are, with an open hearted and **non-judgemental attitude**. This is a process of observing thoughts, emotions and sensations as they come and go, with an attitude of curiosity and acceptance.

Mindfulness is more than learning to pay attention – it also implies cultivating an attitude of openness, interest and acceptance. When we fight with the thoughts and feelings we would rather not be having we actually feed them with more attention and increase the impact that they have. So learning to notice them and be non-reactive and non-judgemental of them is an important aspect of learning to be free of them.

Mindfulness can be applied to experiencing everyday activities such as eating, walking, washing the dishes and having a shower. Practising mindfulness can help us to be less caught up in stress, worry and low mood by helping us to develop a greater capacity to engage in our lives by being more fully present. Mindfulness is a skill that can be developed with practice over time.

Combining the skill of mindfulness with the regular practice of meditation involves intentionally **placing our attention on the breath**, and observing each rise and fall of the breath. It is natural that our minds will not stay aware of the breath for very long. The mind will inevitably wander off and soon we will be thinking or planning or worrying. The practice of mindfulness is to **be aware when our attention has wandered**, and then, without judgement, gently but firmly redirect our attention back to the breath.

At the beginning of practice it is likely that our minds will wander many, many times. While this can be frustrating, it is important to remember that the moment we are aware that our mind has wandered, we are practising mindfulness. Then we simply return our attention to observing the breath, again and again and again.

Health TIP . . . .

If you are finding it difficult to practise mindfulness meditation on your own consider downloading a guided mindfulness exercise.

How To Meditate Mindfully

Days can roll into one without punctuation. When this happens life becomes a blur. It is important that we pause throughout the day to remind ourselves to be aware and mindful. A way to do this is to practise the two exercises below frequently throughout the day[3].

The 'full stop' could be practised any time from 5-30 minutes twice a day depending on motivation and opportunity, and the 'comma' for 15 seconds-2 minutes as often as you remember throughout the day. The comma is particularly useful between having completed one activity and beginning another.

EXERCISE 1 – 'THE FULL STOP'[3]

Sit in a chair so that your spine is upright and balanced but relaxed. Have your body symmetrical and allow your eyes to gently close. Now, move the attention gently through each step. Be conscious of your body and its connection with the chair. Feel your feet on the floor. Notice if your feet are tense. If so, allow them to relax if they want to. Similarly,

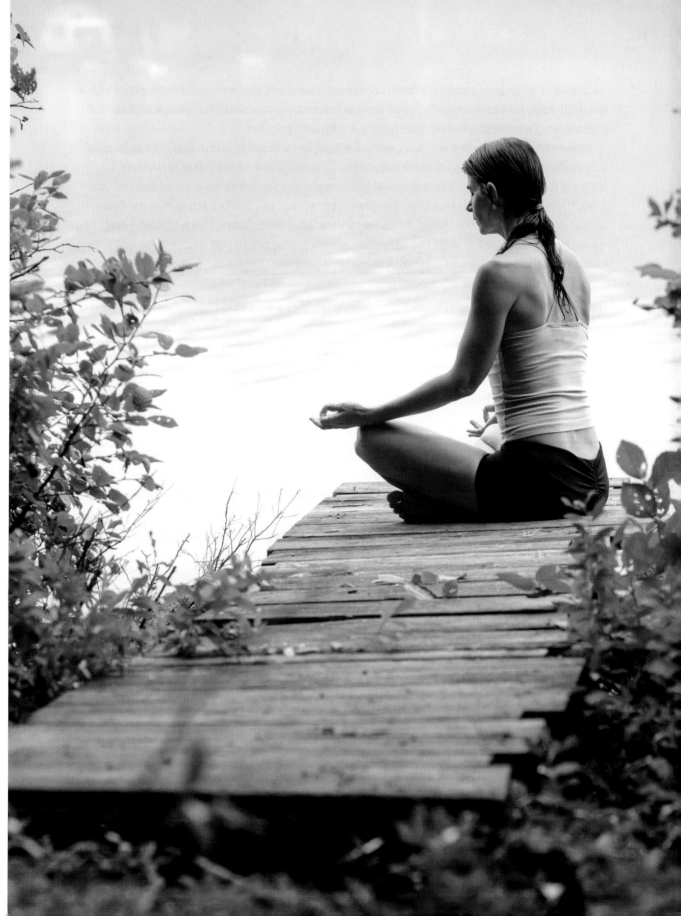

boost oxytocin, the bonding hormone

Oxytocin is the hormone of love and bonding. It is a hormone that is released from a part of our brains called the pituitary gland during those special, close moments with people we love such as during breastfeeding, childbirth, and even during orgasm. It allows us to bond with loved ones and makes us feel good. It also allows us to trust and connect with others. Sadly many individuals do not experience the positive benefits of oxytocin due to social isolation, lack of meaningful relationships, or due to other life circumstances that have resulted in them being distanced from others. Yet studies have revealed that good health is directly connected with the quality of social connections that we have[1] and the quality of our social connections is related to how much oxytocin our brains release during our interactions with those significant others[2].

Many people experience poor health because they are lonely, and they long for someone to share life's experiences with. I have noticed this to be true even for those individuals who eat well, exercise, and do all the other 'right' things when it comes to healthy living. If they are devoid of positive social and emotional connections they suffer in some way, whether it is from unexplained physical symptoms or mental health problems.

I recall a beautiful woman in her forties who came to see me as a patient struggling with a general feeling of being unwell. She suffered from fatigue, headaches, stomach pains, and an inability to sleep. We undertook many investigations to get to the root cause of her issues and found that she had a clean bill of physical health. There was simply no obvious physical explanation for her symptoms. Over the course of several consultations she revealed that she was desperately lonely. She had never been in a longstanding relationship because she suffered with very low self-confidence. This stemmed from being put down by a high-school boyfriend due to her mild cerebral palsy she had suffered at birth. The emotional drain from feeling so alone was affecting her physically. I suggested some counselling to deal with her underlying feelings of inadequacy and low self-esteem to which she was agreeable. She found that over the course of treatment her confidence levels began to rise and she started to date again. As a result, her mood lifted and so did her well-being.

This story highlights the fact that in order for us to truly realise the benefits of healthy living on our physical and mental well-being we also need to have positive social interactions. This does not just mean intimate relationships but also friendships. In essence we need to be socially connected in order to be well.

Let us expand on the health benefits of having social connections and then look at how we can form these strong connections and maximise oxytocin release in our brains.

Social Connections & Good Health

Interestingly, developing strong connections has been shown to be as effective as diet and exercise in determining health and well-being[1]. Scientists have suggested that the reason for this is because social interaction is hardwired into our brains and is needed for survival[3].

Health TIP . . . .

The quality of our health is directly linked to the quality of our relationships.

In fact, having social connections has been shown to reduce many of the following major diseases and health conditions[3,4]:

- Heart disease
- High blood pressure
- Stroke
- Depression
- Anxiety
- Cognitive decline
- Vulnerability to infection
- Chronic pain
- Type 2 diabetes in men
- Obesity
- Cancer
- Insomnia
- Death

The reduction of the above conditions has been shown to occur regardless of a person's social status, age, gender or race[4]. This means that our need for connectedness is universal, as is evidenced by examining all cultures from around the world.

Furthermore, studies have repeatedly revealed that those of us who are highly socially connected, have good social support, and have rewarding social relationships report more overall well-being, improved self-esteem, less anxiety and fewer depressive symptoms, less social avoidance, and less sensitivity to being rejected[3].

But it can be difficult to develop true friendships in a society that values personal autonomy, anonymity and independence. We have such busy lifestyles that many of us find ourselves socially isolated. I have heard it said that the way we live today is like living in 'social Siberia', meaning we exist in such close proximity to others but are so far away in terms of emotional connection. So, that being said, how do you develop and maintain positive social connections?

How To Build Positive Social Connections

Firstly, studies have suggested that it is the quality and not the quantity of relationships that determines whether we feel that we are socially connected. So focussing on developing a small number of meaningful friendships is a better approach than trying to be friends with everyone.

Secondly, forming relationships is about developing mutual areas of interest. So participating in a joint hobby or cause can lead to lifelong friendships. Examples might be a sporting club, volunteer organisation, church group or other hobby group. Forming friendships based on unhealthy habits such as friends who only meet if alcohol is involved may not be the best approach for forging meaningful and healthy relationships.

Thirdly, developing friendships takes time and effort. Sacrifice is therefore sometimes needed on our behalf as there are so many things competing for our time and attention these days. Investing in quality friendships is like investing in blue-chip shares; the return on investment may not happen straight away but they definitely pay dividends well into the future. In other words, by investing in meaningful friendships we will experience mutual support and long-term benefits. Finally, the health and emotional benefits of having friendships extends to that of the furry kind. Those who own pets on average experience better health and live up to 5 years longer than non-pet owners[5]. So at the very least, or in addition to our human friends, we could consider getting a pet to improve our well-being.

Now that we know how to build a sense of social connectedness into our lives we need to know how to boost those connections in order to experience the maximum amount of bonding and mutual trust. We need to know what the research says about boosting oxytocin release from our brains when we are interacting with others, as oxytocin is considered the key ingredient in forming close ties.

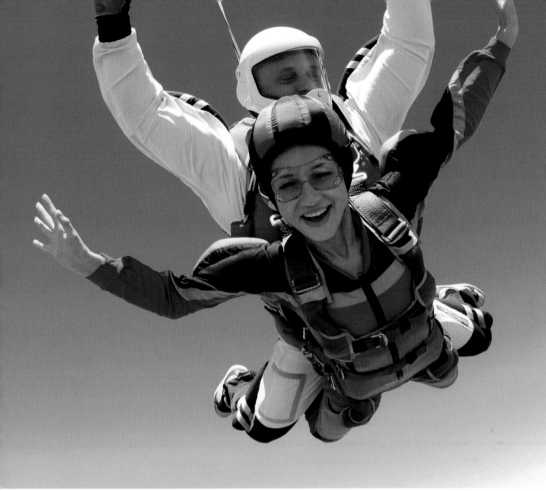

How To Boost Your Oxytocin Levels

According to Paul Zak, neuroeconomist at Claremont Graduate University, California, and author of the book *The Moral Molecule*, there are several ways proven by research to raise oxytocin release[2].

These include the following activities that can be undertaken with a partner, family member, or a friend:

Listen with your eyes. Give the person you are trying to connect with your full, undivided attention.

Give them a gift. Receiving gifts raises oxytocin. The key is not to expect a gift in return, just surprise someone for no reason.

Share a meal together. Sharing a meal releases oxytocin and is therefore a mutually bonding experience.

Meditate while focussing on others. A form of meditation called 'metta', in which one focusses on loving others, is better at fostering social connections than standard mindfulness meditation.

Ride a roller coaster or jump out of an airplane together. Many activities that are moderately stressful and done with one or more other people raise oxytocin. Sharing an adrenaline-raising experience with someone else creates stronger bonding.

Use the 'L' word. Tell those around you that you love them. Oxytocin is the love molecule so it is part of our biochemistry to love others. Saying the words 'I Love You' helps others to express the same.

Hug. Physical touch raises oxytocin, so instead of a handshake try hugging someone instead.

Take Home Points

Our health is directly linked with how socially connected we are.

- The ability to form quality social connections is linked to the release of oxytocin from our brains.
- It is the quality and not the quantity of relationships that determines our level of connection with others and, in turn, the benefits to our health.
- Forming strong connections with others depends on our ability to find areas of mutual interest and to sacrifice time and energy.
- Further strengthening our bond with others may be achieved by raising oxytocin levels through, for example, sharing a meal, giving others our full attention, appropriate physical contact such as a hug, and giving somebody a gift.
- The more our brains get used to releasing oxytocin the easier we will find connecting with significant others. This means that if we get in to the practice of making strong friendships and relationships we will find this will eventually come naturally.

YOUR *Weekly* CHALLENGE . . . .

This week your challenge is to practise forming strong connections with others. This does not have to mean a multitude of different people but focus on strengthening those relationships you already have. Perhaps share a meal with someone, give them a gift or a hug, or even just sit down face to face and give them your undivided attention. These activities all forge strong bonds through the release of oxytocin.

practise the art of letting go

M any people do not realise what a burden not forgiving is until they finally let go. Holding on to a major grudge can lead to a range of emotional, mental and physical health problems. One particular emotion that is often suppressed when holding on to a long-standing grudge, resentment or lack of forgiveness is anger. This suppressed anger can lead to low-grade, underlying and often subconscious chronic stress in your life, which in turn can lead to significant health consequences.

Health FACT

Research has found that 61 per cent of cancer patients have trouble forgiving with over ½ of them reporting very strong difficulties with forgiving[1].

Some of these health consequences may include stress ulcers, heart disease, headaches, insomnia, anxiety, and depression. In addition, author of *The Forgiveness Project*, Dr Michael Barry, has proposed from research that the emotions created by long-term unforgiveness supress the cancer-fighting cells in the body[1].

With this in mind it is important that we first identify in our lives whether or not forgiving someone in a specific situation may be affecting our physical and mental health. This can sometimes be difficult to identify as we may have held a particular grudge unknowingly for many years before it comes to the surface.

I remember a time in my adolescence when I was bullied by a group of girls at a new school I had attended. Their taunts wounded my feelings and self-confidence. What I did not realise is that these feelings led to some deep-seated anger and insecurity in general.

This I carried around like a hidden sore and was surprised to feel exactly the same level of intense emotion come to the surface when I happened to bump into one of these bullies many years later. Not wanting to be ruled by old emotional scars and not wanting to give my power over to someone else I made a decision to forgive those girls who were now women. The sense of lightness I felt was amazing. But in order to forgive, first I had to understand what forgiveness truly is and what it is not.

What Is Forgiveness?

Forgiveness is difficult to define and may look different for everyone. The American Psychological Association describes forgiveness generally as, '... a process or the result of a process that involves a change in emotion and attitude regarding an offender.'[2] This process is considered intentional and voluntary and driven by a deliberate decision to forgive. The end result of forgiveness is a decrease in motivation to retaliate towards others or maintain your distance from those you have held unforgiveness towards despite their actions. It requires letting go of negative emotions towards them and may involve replacing those negative emotions with feelings of compassion and wanting to do a kind act towards that person/s.

Forgiveness may involve reconciliation or restoration of a relationship with that person who hurt you, or it may occur independent to this. Forgiveness can be one-sided and does not necessarily involve the other person accepting fault or offering you their forgiveness if they feel wronged by you as well.

Forgiveness, however, is not:

• Condoning - failing to see the action as wrong and in need of forgiveness

• Excusing - not holding the person or group responsible for the action

• Pardoning - stopping the pursuit of justice for wrong actions

• Forgetting - removing awareness of the offence from consciousness i.e. to forgive is more than just not thinking about the offence

There is a process to forgiveness and once a decision is made that you are going to forgive someone and not allow resentment towards them steal your joy, peace and health, then you are ready to start along the pathway to forgiveness.

So Why Should We Forgive?

There are some real benefits to forgiveness, which have nothing to do with the person you are forgiving. There may be some secondary sense of relief and possibly restoration of a relationship between you and the other person who has hurt you, but the reason you forgive is not because you owe them but because forgiveness is in your best interests. So what are some of the benefits of forgiveness?

A summary research paper collated by the American Psychological Association on forgiveness states that forgiving someone has the following benefits[2]:

- Aids psychological healing through positive changes in affect
- Improves physical and mental health
- Restores a forgiver's sense of personal power
- Helps bring about reconciliation between the offended and offender
- Promotes hope for future relationships and situations

What Is The Best Way to Forgive?

As suggested by psychologist Dr Michael Barry, the process of forgiveness may involve following 4 steps[1]. Keep in mind that the first 3 steps do not have to be completed in any order but the end result of forgiveness is always the final step, which is to let go.

- Express the emotion
- Understand why
- Rebuild safety
- Let go

Express the emotion: Whatever the crime or injustice or violation, you need to fully express how it made you feel. Those feelings, whether they be hurt, pain or anger need to be deeply felt and expressed. If it is possible to express it to the person who has hurt you, great, but if not a proxy such as an empty chair, a heartfelt letter, or just yelling into a pillow may suffice.

Understand why: Our brain will continue to search for some explanation until it is satisfied. We may not agree with the reasoning behind why someone did what they did, and it may be completely opposite to the way we would have acted. Nevertheless, our brain needs to make sense of why the act took place. In some situations, even an acceptance of randomness can be a sufficient answer.

Rebuild safety: In order to completely forgive we need to feel a reasonable amount of assurance the act will not recur. Whether it comes in the form of a sincere apology from those who have hurt us, a stronger boundary of defence against that person's behaviour, or removal from that person's influence, safety needs to be re-acquired.

These 3 elements to the forgiveness process help us process the event. They lead to the last step, which is often the most difficult.

Let go: Letting go is making a promise not to hold a grudge. In addition, letting go is making a promise to yourself that you will stop dwelling, replaying or ruminating on the injustice. If letting go feels impossible, it is probably because the first 3 steps in the forgiveness process were not sufficiently completed.

Where Can You Go for Further Help?

If you feel that holding on to unforgiveness towards someone or a group of people is causing you to have poor mental or physical health then consider speaking to a counsellor to undertake forgiveness therapy. This branch of therapy is particularly helpful for those who have been greatly hurt by someone else such as in the case of trauma, abuse or addiction. This is not to say that you cannot start the forgiveness process by yourself but sometimes a supportive and safe place to share your emotions will expedite the healing process. Consider, too, the words of Mahatma Gandhi, '...the weak can never forgive. Forgiveness is an attribute of the strong.'

Take Home Points

Holding on to unforgiveness can harm our health.

- Forgiveness usually involves a 4-step process: express the emotion, understand why, rebuild safety, and finally let go.
- Forgiveness is a deliberate decision and one that we make based on our desire to be mentally and physically released of the pressure and stress of holding on to a grudge.
- Forgiveness does not mean that those who have hurt us are free to walk all over us or to continue to hurt us, but it does mean that they are free to live their lives, as are we, without any feelings of resentment.
- In cases where there is deep-seated unforgiveness in our lives we may benefit from seeing a counsellor to engage in some forgiveness therapy.

YOUR *Weekly* CHALLENGE . . . .

This week your challenge is to practise the art of letting go. Talk to your health practitioner or to a counsellor this week if you feel that unforgiveness is holding you back. Consider writing down a list of those who you are yet to forgive and pick one of these people to start the forgiveness process with. Remember that holding on to a grudge or resentment only continues to hurt us and potentially harm our health.

laugh more

Laughter really is good medicine. When was the last time you had a really good belly laugh? Laughter has been shown not only to be good for you but to be contagious. Have you ever found yourself laughing with someone just because they were laughing? It was as if their laugh was infectious and despite not actually knowing what they were laughing about, your bout of unrestrained amusement left you feeling great! This is the basis of a form of therapy known as 'Laughter Yoga'.

During a session of Laughter Yoga, which is held all over the country, a group of participants meet and literally engage in side-splitting, belly-burning laughter. The verdict from participants is unanimous, '...a strangely liberating and uplifting experience.' Well, as it says in Proverbs 19:22, 'A cheerful heart *is* good medicine.'

Studies have shown that laughter offers one of the most powerful and natural healing methods without any side effects. According to a recent study by cardiologists at the University of Maryland Medical Center in Baltimore, laughter, along with an active sense of humour, may help protect you against a heart attack[1]. This study is the first to indicate that laughter may help prevent heart disease.

Furthermore, a group of professors from the University of California, Los Angeles, established the Humor Research Task Force to look into the effects of humour and laughter[2]. Their research indicated that laughter can help:

- Reduce stress and elevate mood
- Foster instant relaxation
- Lower blood pressure
- Boost the immune system
- Improve brain functioning
- Protect the heart

- Connect you to others
- Increase your pain-tolerance level

Laughter may also extend your life. A large study of 54 000 Norwegians, undertaken at the Norwegian University of Science and Technology, showed that those who have a sense of humour outlive those who don't find life funny; and the survival edge is particularly evident for people with cancer[3]. That is, cancer sufferers who retain their sense of humour have a higher survival rate than those who do not. Some of the most resilient patients I have had the pleasure of treating in the past have been those who have maintained a sense of humour about their situation.

Health FACT . . . .

Children on average laugh 200 times per day whilst adults generally only laugh around 15 times per day[4].

Interestingly, research conducted at the University of California also suggests that a sense of humor can bring families closer together[4]. Apparently laughing together is a way to connect, and a good sense of humor also can make kids smarter, healthier and better able to cope with challenges. Apparently, a sense of humour is not necessarily just part of our genetic make-up, like blue eyes or the colour of our hair. A sense of humor is actually a learnt quality that can be developed in children, rather than something they're born with. Furthermore, kids with a well-developed sense of humor are happier and more optimistic, have higher self-esteem, and can handle differences well. Kids who can appreciate and share humour are better liked by their peers and more able to handle the adversities of childhood such as bullying.

Why Is Laughter So Good For You?

The positive effects of laughter are attributed to powerful chemicals released in the brain called 'endorphins'. These are stronger than any artificial painkiller. Endorphins also trigger a positive feeling in the body, similar to that of morphine. For example, the feeling that follows a run or workout is often described as 'euphoric'. That feeling, known as a 'runner's high', can be accompanied by a positive and energising outlook on life.

How Much Laughing Should You Be Doing?

Apparently, all that is needed to gain the benefits of these little powerhouse chemicals is 10 hearty laughs per day[5]. This comes naturally for children, who apparently laugh on

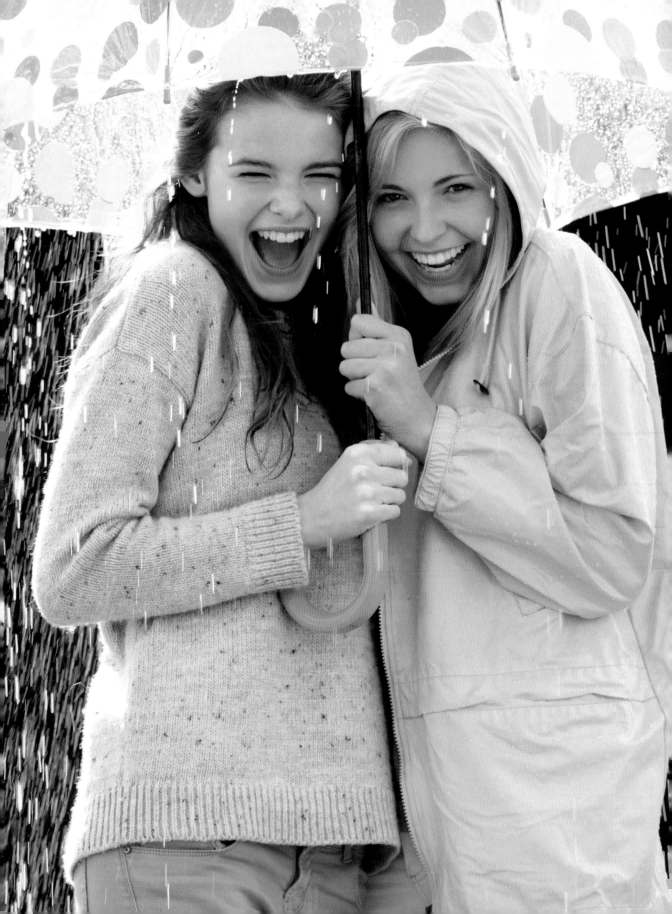

average 200 times per day[4]. Whilst the average adult laughs a lot less than this at an average of 15 times per day[4]. At what point do we start to take life so seriously? Perhaps when responsibilities start creeping up, when aches and pains start creeping in, and when life just seems too hard. But that is where laughter, even if it is feigned outbursts of joy, can help us to overcome life's challenges. Perhaps try to incorporate some belly laughs into your day. May I suggest watching a comedy on occasion, go out of your way to remember jokes to share with others, learn to enjoy the company of those annoyingly happy people, and most of all let us learn to laugh at ourselves and life more often.

Health TIP

Laughter really is the best medicine. Try and have 10 belly laughs per day.

Take Home Points

Laughter is the best medicine
- Those who laugh often have been found to live longer, have greater survival from cancer, lower blood pressure, less depression, stronger hearts and better immune systems.
- Laughter is infectious. Consider associating yourself with someone who laughs a lot.
- Sense of humour is in-built but can also be learnt and be developed.
- Of all the traits that are admired in a spouse, sense of humour ranks as in the top 5.
- Laughter connects families and can help children handle bullying.
- Laughing releases endorphins, which are our natural painkillers.
- Consider doing something fun and watching something funny often.
- Learn to laugh at life and laugh at yourself more often.

YOUR *Weekly* CHALLENGE

This week your challenge is to laugh more. Consider hiring out a funny movie and watching it with friends. Develop your sense of humour this week by remembering jokes to share with others, laugh often at yourself and the sometimes lunacy of life, and even practise laughing until it becomes a learnt habit like any other.

recognise allergies

Allergies are becoming more and more common with around 1 in 3 people suffering from some sort of allergy[1]. Yet I have found in clinical practice that quite often people do not realise they are allergic to something that is causing recurrent and sometimes debilitating symptoms. A typical example of this is dustmite or mould allergy. The only symptom you might notice is fatigue and headache or a postnasal drip that just does not seem to go away. Because allergies are so common and can cause significant health problems it is worth discussing how you can recognise if you have an allergy and also learn what you can do about it. Note that food intolerance is not discussed here as it is covered in Simple Health Habit #24 on recognising food upsets.

Health FACT . . . .

1 in 3 Australian adults will suffer from **allergies at some stage in their lives**[1].

Why Do Allergies Happen?

Allergies occur when your immune system overreacts to a usually harmless substance. This substance, called an 'allergen', can be anything, but some things are frequently found to cause allergic reactions. Most occur shortly after exposure to an allergen. For example, seasonal allergies are likely to worsen on the same day that the pollen count goes up. If you are allergic to cats and you visit the home of someone who owns a cat, you are likely to start developing an allergic reaction before you leave the house. However some allergic reactions can occur hours or days after exposure to an allergen e.g. some forms of contact dermatitis to plants can develop several days after the exposure.

Allergies can develop at any time in our lives but are most common in our childhood years due to our developing immune system. It is possible to go through life and not be allergic to anything; at the other end of the spectrum, some people develop allergies to multiple substances. There is a genetic component to the development of allergic tendencies. However you do not necessarily develop an allergy to the same substances as your relatives.

Why Are Allergies So Common?

We do not yet know what is causing allergies to become so common. There have been many theories proposed including the 'hygiene hypothesis', which states that we live in a society that is too clean and this is preventing people from developing proper immunity. Other theories centre around our food not being the same as it used to be. Artificial colours, preservatives, flavours and pesticides are blamed. Others state it is an imbalance between omega-6 and omega-3 fats in our diet that is causing more allergies, or perhaps a change in the microbes that live in our gut that is responsible. Unfortunately at this stage in our understanding of why allergies develop we are left with a big question mark. Hopefully with advances in research we will know more in the coming years.

What Can You Develop Allergies to?

Common substances that people can be allergic to include:

- Dustmites
- Pollen
- Mould
- Latex
- Medications
- Plants
- Cat, dog and horse dander (hair)
- Chemicals

I have even met patients who have been allergic to their own sweat, to the heat, and to contact with their own skin. They develop an itchy rash, welts, and in some cases nausea and a mild fever. These types of allergies are, luckily, rare but they can be very difficult to manage.

What Are the Symptoms of Allergies?

Symptoms of allergies can range from mild to severe and in the case of anaphylaxis can be fatal. Symptoms depend on the allergy, but may include:

- Sneezing
- Runny nose
- Postnasal drip
- Itchy throat
- Dark circles under the eyes
- Red, watery and itchy eyes
- Wheezing
- Coughing
- Breathing problems
- Headache
- Skin rash
- Stomach pains
- Vomiting and diarrhoea

Another common symptom is fatigue. I recall a patient who was waking every morning feeling exhausted. She often cleared her throat and frequently suffered from a sore throat. On further questioning she informed me that she would wake in the middle of the night with a dry mouth and needed to have a glass of water beside her bed. This is a classic symptom of mouth breathing and is commonly associated with dustmite allergy. Dustmites live in bedding and feed off our dead skin cells. In those who are not allergic they cause no problem, but for those of us who react to dustmites going to bed can be problematic. When we discovered what her problem was and reduced her dustmite exposure, her symptoms greatly improved. In particular she is no longer waking exhausted. If you can relate to any of these symptoms it is worth speaking to your health-care practitioner about the possibility of a dustmite allergy.

Should You Have Allergy Testing?

The answer is yes, there is accurate allergy testing available in Australia.

Skin prick tests Selected allergens are applied to the forearm or the back with a dropper, and the skin gently pricked with a sterile lancet. A positive result shows as a red weal or flare on the skin within 20 minutes.

Blood test These tests are useful when skin testing is not possible or is inconclusive. Your GP is able to order this type of testing.

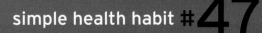

simple health habit #47

get some sunshine

The majority of all living things require sunshine and we are no exception. There is a reason we tend to feel happier on a sunny day – our cells respond to the sun's rays. There has been a lot of concern in the last 3-4 decades about sun exposure and the risk of skin cancer, so much so that we are living year round mostly indoors and if we do venture out in the sun we tend to be almost completely covered up. So what is so important about being exposed to sunshine and how can we ensure that we are exposing our skin to the sun's rays in the safest way possible?

The Healing Power of Sunshine

There are numerous health benefits associated with exposure to sunshine, including[1]:

- Boosting vitamin D levels.
- Enhancing mood and energy through the release of endorphins – some people are so affected when they are not exposed to sunshine for prolonged periods that they develop a severely depressed mental and physical state called Seasonal Affective Disorder (SAD). This is particularly a problem in countries that experience little sunshine for many months of the year. The treatment for SAD is light therapy. A milder condition can occur in Australia where individuals do not see the sun for most of the daylight hours due to working for long periods indoors.
- Treating skin diseases, such as psoriasis, vitiligo, atopic dermatitis and scleroderma.
- Setting our body clock and improving sleep.
- Relieving pain from fibromyalgia, a chronic autoimmune condition.
- Inducing nitric oxide (NO) release in the body, which helps protect your skin against UV damage, offers cardiovascular protection, promotes wound healing through its antimicrobial effect, and has some anti-cancer benefits.
- Protecting against and suppressing symptoms of multiple sclerosis (MS).

healthy habits: 52 ways to better health

Of these, the most topical at the moment is vitamin D and the important role it plays in our health. Let us look at this briefly before we look at how much sunshine exposure we need each day.

The Importance of Vitamin D

We are currently experiencing an epidemic of vitamin D deficiency. At least ⅓ of Australians are vitamin D deficient[2]. Interestingly, studies have suggested that vitamin D should not really be considered a vitamin at all, since it behaves more like a hormone in the body. That is, it is made in the skin, gets into your bloodstream and then goes into the liver and the kidney where it becomes activated as a key steroid hormone called Calcitriol. It then goes to the intestines, bones and other tissues, affecting metabolic pathways and the expression of a myriad genes.

Vitamin D's active form interacts with almost every cell in the body directly or indirectly, potentially targeting up to 2000 genes, or about 6 per cent of the human genome. It is necessary for numerous cellular functions, and when the body does not have what it needs to function optimally, it follows that we can experience a decline in health and put ourselves at risk of disease.

Some of the conditions associated with vitamin D deficiency include[3]:

- Osteoporosis (weakened bones) in older adults as vitamin D controls calcium levels in the body
- Bone and muscle pain
- Rickets (softened bones) in children
- Multiple sclerosis
- Diabetes (type 1 and type 2)
- Various types of cancers (particularly colon cancer)
- Heart disease
- Mental health conditions (including schizophrenia and depression)
- Worse outcomes in stroke
- Altered immunity and other autoimmune diseases

Although there is a strong link that these conditions are associated with vitamin D deficiency, more research is needed to determine whether optimising vitamin D levels will prevent these conditions.

What Factors Affect Your Vitamin D Levels?

Vitamin D is primarily made from exposure of the skin to ultraviolet type B (UVB) light but also depends upon the health of your gut, kidney and liver as these organs are also involved in the production of the active form of vitamin D, Calcitriol. Where you live, your skin type, the current climate and your overall health will determine how much vitamin D you make.

The lowest vitamin D levels are found in individuals who:

Live at High Latitudes At higher latitudes, the amount of vitamin D-producing UVB light reaching the earth's surface goes down in the winter because of the low angle of the sun.

Live in Colder Climates Skin that is warm is a more efficient producer of vitamin D than skin that is cool. So, on a sunny, hot summer day, you will make more vitamin D than on a cool one.

Cover Up Always Those who burn easily, who have had skin cancer, or who are sensitive to the sun for other reasons will often cover up at all times of the day. Although this is understandable there are safe ways to get enough sun exposure to make vitamin D without putting your skin at risk (as explained below). Continuously applying sunscreen theoretically reduces your vitamin D production but in practice few people apply enough sunscreen frequently enough to affect vitamin D levels.

Work Indoors Office workers and nightshift workers and others who do not get outside much are at risk of vitamin D deficiency.

Have Darker Skin The pigment in skin (melanin) acts as a filter to UVB radiation and reduces the amount of vitamin D that the body makes. As a result, dark-skinned people tend to require more UVB exposure than light-skinned people to generate the same amount of vitamin D. Because I have olive skin I find it near impossible to get enough sun to boost my vitamin D levels while working fulltime. For this reason I take a vitamin D supplement (more on this below).

Are Overweight Fat tissue is said to absorb vitamin D and essentially remove it from the bloodstream. So the more fat tissue you have the more likely you are to be vitamin D deficient.

Are Older Older people have lower levels of the substance in the skin that UVB light converts into the vitamin D precursor, and there's experimental evidence that older people are less efficient vitamin D producers than younger people.

Have Gut Diseases The vitamin D that is consumed in food or as a supplement is absorbed in the part of the small intestine immediately downstream from the stomach. Stomach juices, pancreatic secretions, bile from the liver, and the integrity of the wall of the intestines all have some influence on how much of the vitamin is absorbed. Therefore, conditions that affect the gut and digestion, like coeliac disease, chronic pancreatitis, Crohn's disease and cystic fibrosis can reduce vitamin D absorption.

Have Liver or Kidney Disease Some types of liver disease can reduce absorption of vitamin D because of reduction of bile. With other types of liver disease, steps essential to vitamin D metabolism cannot proceed. Levels of the bioactive form of vitamin D tend to track with the health of the kidneys, so in someone with kidney disease, bioactive vitamin D levels decrease as the disease gets worse, and in end-stage kidney disease, the level is undetectable.

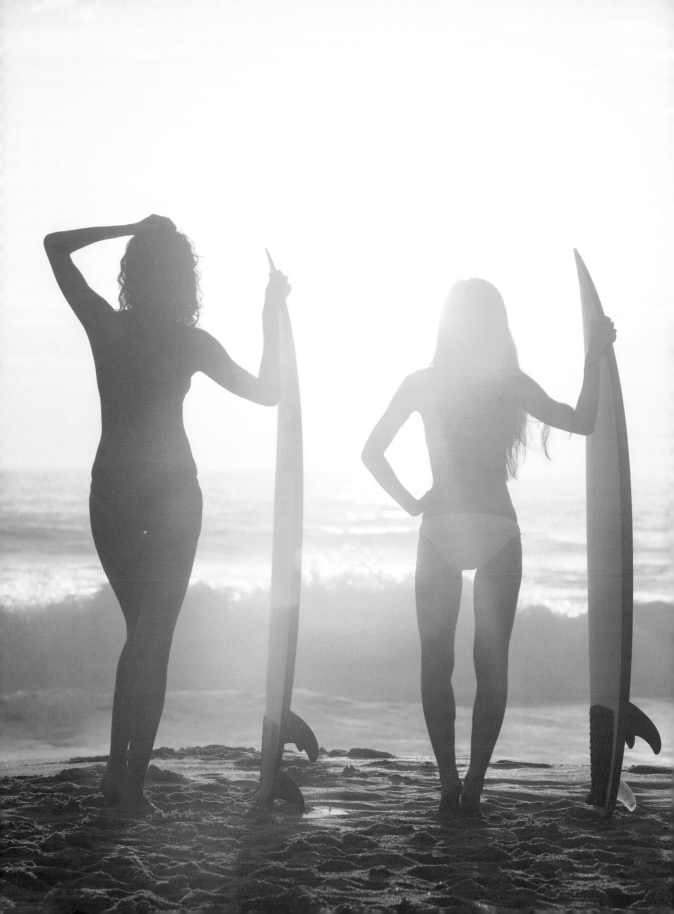

How to Boost Your Vitamin D Levels

Ultraviolet (UV) radiation from the sun is necessary for the production of vitamin D in the skin and is the best natural source of vitamin D. UV radiation from the sun is also the main cause of skin cancer. Unfortunately, Australia is the skin cancer capital of the world. More than 11500 Australian men and women are diagnosed with a melanoma each year, and an estimated 434000 people are treated for one or more non-melanoma skin cancers like basal cell carcinoma (BCC) and squamous cell carcinoma (SCC)[4]. Taking a balanced approach to sun exposure can ensure you get enough vitamin D while minimising your skin cancer risk. Around 10 per cent of vitamin D is also absorbed from certain foods.

Health FACT

Very dark-skinned individuals may require 3 to 6 times as much sun exposure than those who are fair-skinned[3].

The following tips help to safely boost vitamin D levels:

Have a healthy respect for the sun It is a powerful medicine with potentially dangerous side effects for your skin. Treat it like medication, using the lowest dose necessary, but do not avoid it completely. Never fall asleep in the sun.

Always avoid sunburn Repeated sunburn, especially in children and very fair-skinned people, has been linked to melanoma.

Prepare your skin and build up tolerance gradually Start early in the year (spring), or early in the morning before the sun is strongest and slowly build up the amount of time you spend in the sun.

Avoid the hottest part of the day Avoid the midday sun when the risk of sunburn will be the highest. Instead choose to expose your skin in the early morning or late afternoon. Because it is the UV level and not the current outside temperature or presence of full sun that determines risk of sun damage, some people find it helpful to look up the UV index by referring to the Bureau of Meteorology or by downloading a UV Index app on their mobile. When the UV index reaches 3 or higher it is unsafe to be out in the sun. One such app is the SunSmart app.

Expose your skin You will need to expose around 20 per cent of your body to sunlight to absorb enough vitamin D. For example, uncover your face, arms and hands. Always wear sunglasses to protect your eyes from sun damage.

Get around 15-30 minutes of unprotected sun exposure 2-4 times a week Each of us have different needs for unprotected sun exposure to maintain adequate levels of Vitamin D. Depending on your age, what type of skin you have, where you live and what time of the day and year it is, your needs will vary. The farther you live from the equator, the more exposure to the sun you need in order to generate vitamin D. Also, people with dark skin pigmentation may need 20-30 times as much exposure to sunlight as fair-skinned people to generate the same amount of vitamin D. The table below provides a guide to the amount of sun exposure needed (in minutes) in Australia for a fair-skinned person in both summer and winter in different localities.

REGION	SUMMER	WINTER
Cairns	6-7	9-12
Brisbane	6-7	15-19
Sydney	6-8	26-28
Melbourne	6-8	32-52
Adelaide	5-7	25-38
Perth	5-6	20-28
Hobart	7-9	40-47

Adapted from reference 5

Get frequent, short exposures Regular short exposures have been found to be much more effective and safer than intermittent long ones. Note that you cannot generate vitamin D when sitting behind a glass window because the UVB rays necessary for vitamin D production are absorbed by glass.

After your sunscreen-free time in the sun, you must protect yourself If you are going to be out in the sun for longer periods, wear a hat to protect your face and light-coloured clothing that blocks the sun and keeps you cool. If you are looking for a sunscreen with fewer chemicals refer online to Environmental Working Group's list of safer sunscreens[6].

Do not rely on food alone for your vitamin D needs It is almost impossible to meet your vitamin D needs with food alone. Fatty wild-caught fish (not farmed), like salmon and mackerel are the best food sources, as well as eggs, but you would have to eat huge quantities of them daily to get anywhere near what your body needs. Although fortified milk and orange juice do contain vitamin D, you would have to drink at least 10 glasses of each daily to get enough vitamin D.

Take Vitamin D3 supplements if necessary If you do not get enough sun exposure or if your vitamin D blood levels are known to be low, you can supplement with at least 2 000 IU a day of vitamin D3. Often, if you are very deficient, at least 5 000 IU of vitamin D3 will be required. It is best to speak to your doctor before supplementing to make sure you actually need this.

I recommend having your vitamin D blood levels checked once per year. The best time to have them checked, in my opinion, is at the end of summer as your highest vitamin D level is likely to be recorded at that time of year. Vitamin D levels then typically decline to a trough in winter. So if your vitamin D levels are low in summer they will be very low in winter. There is some debate as to what is considered optimal blood vitamin D levels. To prevent disease, it has been suggested to keep vitamin D levels above 50 ng/mL, yet other studies have reported that more optimal levels for health are around 75-110 ng/mL[7].

Take Home Points

Sunshine is very important for health and well-being.

- Exposure to sun on a regular basis may help to prevent osteoporosis, depression, diabetes, body aches and pains, MS and other autoimmune conditions.
- One of the major benefits to getting some sunshine exposure regularly is production of vitamin D, an important hormone-like substance that has numerous functions in the body.
- In Australia we have epidemic proportions of vitamin D deficiency.
- One reason for this is that many of us are afraid to be exposed to the sun due to skin cancer risk. Many of us are also working more indoors and do not have adequate, regular exposure to direct sunlight.
- In order to make enough vitamin D we need around 15-30 minutes of sunlight exposure per day, several times per week, depending on the time of year, our location, and our skin type.
- Avoid the hottest part of the day and look out for a UV index of less than 3, which is safe for exposure.
- Avoid getting sunburnt, which increases the risk of skin cancer, especially in fair-skinned individuals and in children.
- Consider having your vitamin D levels checked annually at around the end of summer and supplement if necessary with a vitamin D3 liquid or tablet.

YOUR *Weekly* CHALLENGE . . . .

This week your challenge is to boost your vitamin D levels by getting enough sun exposure. Consider, too, having your vitamin D levels tested by your doctor.

love the skin
you are in

Our skin is one of the most important organs in our body. Much of the time we do not view our skin as an organ but it is in fact a metabolically active part of our body just as much as any other organ. In fact, our skin is the largest organ we have and functions to protect us from our outside environment, to house our peripheral nervous system so that we can sense our environment, and to provide a casing around our other body structures so that we can interact with our environment safely. It is composed of numerous different cells – from skin cells to immune cells to blood and nerve cells. Our skin is also a great reflector of our internal health.

Health FACT . . . .

Our skin cells are said to completely renew in 7 year cycles. That means you have the opportunity to greatly improve your skin health in this time.

When we are lacking in certain nutrients or suffering from some level of disease our skin can start to show signs of this. So much so that the health of our skin is not just skin deep but very much in tune with the rest of our body. It is also an organ that needs a great deal of nutrients to be healthy but can receive the least by way of sacrifice to provide the rest of the body first. Remember, too, that hair and nails are just an extension of our skin and so these structures can also be affected when our nutritional balance or health in general is not sound. The result is that our external picture to the world is not one of health and radiance. As a doctor I am trained to notice first someone's skin, nails, and to some extent hair; they can signal the level of internal body health. You can always tell someone who is in good health versus someone who is not by the health of these structures. So what are the things to watch out for when looking at your skin, nails and hair? What are the poor health indicators?

Beauty Is More than Skin Deep

Some of the signs of poor skin health include:

- Dry skin
- Itchy and inflamed skin
- Rashes
- Pigmentation
- Loss of skin colouring
- Flaky skin or hair
- Pimples, pustules, boils, and other skin sores
- Cracked skin
- Brittle nails and hair
- Pitting or ridges in your nails
- Spoon shaped nails
- Discoloured nails
- White spots in your nails

All of these conditions can suggest an underlying health condition. When health is sound your skin will glow and not show symptoms as above, your nails will be strong with white tips and pink bases, and your hair will not be brittle but will shine. We can of course ruin the constitution of our nails and hair by way of chemical treatments such as dying, false nails, too frequent washing etc. This is not what I am specifically referring to but rather the condition of your nails, hair and skin in its natural state. So what can result in reduced health of our skin, hair and nails?

Conditions That Affect the Health of Your Skin, Hair & Nails

The health conditions that can impact on our skin, hair and nails can be broadly classified as nutritional deficiencies, excessive chemical and sun exposure, hormone imbalances, infections, allergies and intolerances and system diseases. These are individually discussed below.

Nutritional Deficiencies Deficiencies in either the intake or absorption of zinc, vitamin C, silica, omega-3 essential fatty acids, as well as antioxidants can greatly impact the health of our skin and can cause poor wound healing, rashes, loss of skin shine and lubrication, and susceptibility to skin infections.

Excessive Chemical Exposure Using harsh skincare and hair and nail products can strip these structures of their natural oils and protective surfacing. Be kind to your skin and avoid over-washing it. Use products that are chemical free, including free of parabens, fragrances, foaming agents, and are slightly acidic in pH. Avoid fake tans that are not based on natural ingredients. Remember that your skin does breathe and so products that are applied to your skin, scalp, and to some degree your nails can be absorbed into your bloodstream.

Excessive Sun Exposure Exposure to ultraviolet light in small amounts is beneficial for our health but in large amounts can cause significant damage to the superficial and deep layers of our skin. This can lead to pigmentation, loss of skin elasticity, wrinkles, and in some cases skin cancer. More on how to safely protect yourself from the sun's rays in the next chapter.

Hormone Imbalances Imbalances of male and female hormones can cause skin conditions such as acne, pigmentation, hair loss or thinning, changes in the elasticity of the skin causing sagging. Excessive stress hormone levels can also cause skin conditions such as itching, pigmentation and poor wound healing.

Skin Infections Certain infections of the skin (as well as nails and hair) whether it be bacterial, viral, or fungal can cause longstanding and sometimes undiagnosed rashes, sores, and itching. Many times these can be easily treated.

Allergies & Intolerances Allergies, from food allergies or something in our environment commonly express themselves in itching of the skin. Eczema and dermatitis are examples. Both of these conditions rely on avoiding the allergic substance in order to have full relief. Food intolerances can also cause eczema-like skin irritations and can be very hard to pinpoint. By eliminating the food responsible, the rash will resolve.

System Diseases Many autoimmune diseases such as lupus, psoriasis, coeliac disease, inflammatory bowel disease, and diabetes can express themselves in some form of skin illness. This can range from rashes to wounds that just will not heal. Diseases of the liver and kidneys, which are the detoxification and filtering organs of the body, respectively, can lead to skin rashes, itchiness, and yellowing or greying of the skin.

How to Properly Diagnose Your Skin Condition

In order to identify where your skin condition may stem from it is important to have it properly looked into. This often involves a blood test, perhaps a painless skin or nail scrapping, or a more invasive skin biopsy. It is important to have this looked into in the early stages of the disease to avoid significant damage to your skin, hair, and nails which can ultimately take much longer to treat.

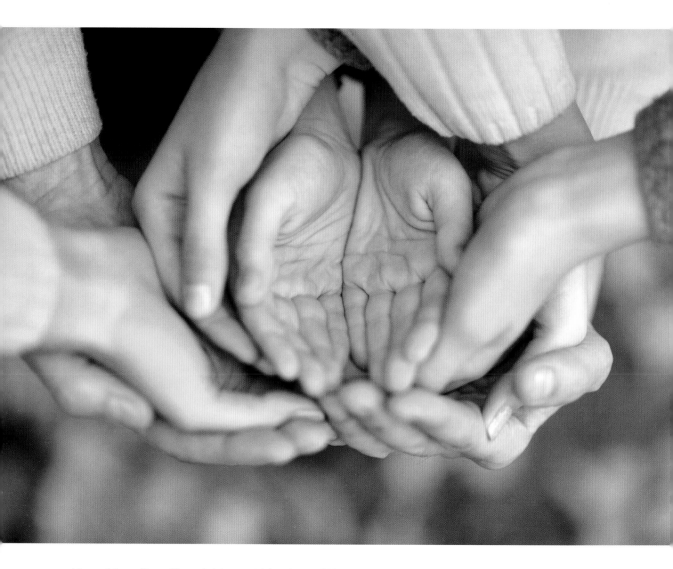

How You Can Treat Your Skin Conditions

The best course of treatment will largely be determined by the cause of the skin condition. Some skin conditions cannot be treated but can be managed. Sometimes skin conditions will come and go throughout a person's life and then one day spontaneously resolve.

Once a cause has been identified then treatment or management can be implemented. Try not to self-diagnose when it comes to skin conditions, or any other condition for that matter, as the causes can be wide and varied and are best diagnosed through the eyes of someone experienced in dealing with skin conditions such as your health professional.

Most people will benefit in terms of skin health from looking after their nutritional intake. This means ensuring you are getting enough zinc, vitamin C, vitamin E, silica, antioxidants and omega-3 fats in your diet and, if not, then consider taking a supplement. Looking after your kidneys by drinking enough water and looking after your liver by avoiding toxin exposure such as alcohol, excessive painkillers, cigarette smoke and food chemicals will also ensure that you have radiant skin.

Our skin is the first point of contact with our environment and the health of our skin can affect our level of well-being and confidence so it is important that we look after it.

Take Home Points

Skin health is more than just skin deep.

- The health of our skin extends to healthy nails and hair, which are just modified skin structures.
- Certain nutritional deficiencies, as well as environmental exposures and system diseases can impact on the health of our skin.
- When we are healthy our skin generally reflects this.
- Healthy skin tends to glow and is free from rashes, flakiness, sores, pigmentation and other irritations.
- Healthy hair is strong and shiny, and healthy nails are smooth and not brittle, chipped or discoloured.
- There are some common nutritional deficiencies that can impact on the health of our skin, hair and nails and these include zinc, vitamin C, vitamin E, silica, antioxidants and omega-3 essential fatty acids.
- Getting enough of these nutrients through food or supplementing with vitamins may greatly improve the condition of our skin, hair and nails.
- It is important that we do not self-diagnose skin conditions as some can be caused by serious illnesses and it is therefore worth having it properly looked into by a trained health professional.

YOUR *Weekly* CHALLENGE . . . .

This week your challenge is to look after your skin (and hair and nails) and recognise whether any skin conditions may be due to common nutritional deficiencies or other causes. Take steps this week to protect your skin and provide it with what it needs to be healthy.

ward off cancer cells

Cancer is, for many people, a frightening word but it does not have to be. Nowadays there are many very effective early detection tests, and diagnosis and treatment options available for cancer. There are also several ways that we can protect our bodies from developing cancer in the first place. Many patients that I come across believe that cancer is not something you can prevent but rather just a matter of chance or genetics, or a combination of both; but this is simply not the case. Let us briefly touch on what cancer actually is.

Health FACT

Over the course of 1 lifetime about every 1:2 males and 1:3 females in most Westernised countries will develop cancer[1]. Many of these cancers can be prevented by lifestyle.

What Is Cancer?

Cancer cells form on a daily basis in all of our bodies and as we age the number of cancer cells being produced increases. This is why cancer occurs more frequently as we get older. The fact that these cancer cells do not always develop into solid tumours is due to our body's natural defences against cancer cells. So cancer cells are just rogue normal body cells that have become mutated in such a way that they become a law unto themselves. They do not follow the usual rules of replication or growth and so take over organ systems and can overwhelm the body. This is why people start to develop secondary cancers in body sites distant to where the original cancer formed; most commonly in the liver, brain, bones and spine. Cancer can initially form in just about every tissue of the body and then spread. So what causes cancer cells to mutate from normal body cells in the first place?

What Causes Cancer?

The most notable substances known to cause mutation of cancer cells in the body are free radicals. Free radicals are highly reactive chemicals produced in our bodies during normal cellular function. Much like a bumper car at a fun park banging into other cars, the guard rails, and anything else it comes into contact with, free radicals cause damage to cells, which can lead to DNA changes. When DNA changes, normal body cells can mutate into cancer cells.

This is usually not a problem if the number of free radicals in the body are being neutralised by substances called antioxidants, which are found directly in the food we eat or are produced in the body from food nutrients. The problem arises when there is an imbalance between the numbers of free radicals being produced and the number of antioxidants available in our body to cancel these out. So there are potentially 2 types of situations where free radicals will rule - if the production of free radicals is increased in our body and/or if the number of antioxidants is low. As the table below indicates these situations can occur due to the following:

HIGH LEVELS OF FREE RADICALS	LOW LEVELS OF ANTIOXIDANTS
Toxin Exposure (cigarette smoke, environmental toxins, pesticides, nitrosamines produced from charcoaled, smoked, and processed meats, other potential carcinogenic chemicals)	Poor dietary intake of fresh fruits and vegetables
Radiation Exposure (excessive UV radiation, ionising radiation)	High intake of processed foods
Heavy Metal Exposure	Low sun exposure leading to inadequate vitamin D
High levels of emotional or physical stress incl. excessive amounts of exercise	
Obesity	

Although exposure to the above factors may increase your risk of free radical cell damage this will not necessarily lead to cancer formation. It may depend on the amount of free radical exposure as well as individual differences in the way our bodies deal with free radicals and cell damage. Nevertheless there are some simple strategies we can follow to help reduce our risk of developing cancer.

How to Protect Your Body from Cancer

Below are some suggestions to ward off cancer cells from forming in your body. The more
of these you do the higher your protection against cancer formation.

- Eat plenty of fresh fruits and vegetables that contain antioxidants.
- Choose wholegrains over highly processed grains as wholegrains contain fibre known
  to reduce potential cancer-causing toxins from the bowel[3].
- Avoid artificial sweeteners due to concerns about effects on cancer development.
- Add the spice turmeric to your food as it contains a compound shown to prevent
  cancer known as curcumin[4].
- Drink green tea as studies have indicated that it reduces the risk of developing many
  cancers[5].
- Avoid processed, charcoaled and smoked meats, which produce nitrosamines,
  potential bowel cancer causing compounds[6]. For similar reasons avoid over-browning
  your meat; rather choose to steam, broil, bake or lightly stir-fry.
- Avoid getting sunburnt as UV radiation damage has been linked to the development
  of skin cancer[7]. Interestingly, not getting enough vitamin D can also potentially lead
  to cancer formation as vitamin D acts as an antioxidant[5] (Refer to Simple Health
  Habit #47 for tips on safe sun exposure).
- Wear rubber gloves if using chemicals for cleaning or better still check for natural
  cleaning alternatives and personal care products. Do not use aerosolised air
  fresheners. Instead choose fresh flowers, natural orange spray or scent pots.
- Avoid using non-stick cookwear that is cracked as this can leach toxic chemicals into
  your food[8]. Instead opt to use stainless steel, ceramic or glass.
- Avoid bisphenol-A (BPA) found in many plastic containers, plastic food wrap, water
  bottles and canned foods, as this has been linked to cancer development amongst
  other health concerns[9]. Look for BPA-free varieties or better still store food in glass
  Pyrex or stainless steel containers. Avoid using plastic food wrap or at the very least
  do not heat food in the microwave covered in plastic wrap, and choose stainless steel
  water bottles.
- Practise stress-reduction strategies regularly.

- Quit smoking, which contains at least 40 known cancer-causing chemicals[10].
- Exercise regularly as this has been shown to reduce cancer incidence[11]. Keep in mind that if you are training heavily consider taking an extra dose of antioxidants to buffer the high numbers of free radicals being produced in your body.
- Consider taking an extra antioxidant supplement if you are over the age of 50 years and you do not eat enough fruit and vegetables. Choose one that contains vitamin C, beta-carotene, vitamin D, vitamin E as well as selenium.

Take Home Points

Cancer does not have to be a frightening word.
- There are ways to help protect your body from the development of cancer.
- Many cancers are lifestyle related and are not just a matter of chance or genetics.
- By eating enough fresh fruits, vegetables and wholegrains you can reduce your risk of cancer formation significantly.
- Doing regular exercise as well as getting a little sunlight exposure can help protect against many cancers.
- Avoid unnecessary exposure to potential carcinogens such as BPA-containing plastics, non-stick cookwear, artificial sweeteners and cleaning products or personal care products containing numerous potentially harmful chemicals.
- Other strategies for reducing your risk of cancer formation are to work on stress reduction strategies, stop smoking, and avoid consuming processed, charcoaled or smoked meats.

YOUR *Weekly* CHALLENGE . . . .

This week your challenge is to make some lifestyle changes that reduce the risk of cancer cells forming in your body. Choose at least 1 of the suggestions listed above that you are not already doing.

choose supplements wisely

In today's society it appears you can buy a supplement for just about anything. Pills, powders, potions and various tinctures are widely available that make a variety of health claims. But do these actually work and should everyone be taking a supplement of some description? This is the question I am commonly asked and it is important that we know the answer to avoid harming our bodies or at the very least to avoid unnecessary spending.

What Are Supplements?

Supplements come with different ingredients and different potential health benefits or claims.

These supplements include but are not limited to:

Vitamins - contain either several vitamins in low dose in a multivitamin formulation or come as individual vitamins or groups of vitamins e.g. multi B supplement.

Minerals - contain either several minerals in low dose in a multimineral formulation or come as individual minerals e.g. selenium, zinc, copper etc.

Oils - can be found in capsule or liquid form and include krill oil, cod liver oil, fish oil, and flaxseed oil.

Antioxidants - formulations containing antioxidant compounds such as resveratrol, green tea extract, glutathione, n-acetyl cysteine etc.

Herbal Supplements - include liquid, powder or capsule herbal extracts e.g. vitex, silymarin, horny goat weed etc.

Greens Powders - contain dried green plants including barley grass, spirulina, chlorella and wheatgrass.

Fibre Supplements - soluble and insoluble fibre supplement e.g. psyllium

Protein Powders - contains the protein portion of foods such as whey, rice, pea and soy often mixed with a fibre supplement and a sweetener.

Performance Enhancing Supplements - these include all sport-related supplements such as creatine, L-carnitine, branched chain amino acids, alpha-lipoic acid, d-ribose and glutamine.

Probiotics - contain known strains of beneficial gut bacteria and come in liquid, tablet or powder form.

Health TIP . . . .

Not all supplements suit everyone and not everyone should take supplements. These need to be tailored to individual needs.

Should Everyone Take Supplements?

The general thought that anyone and everyone should take the same supplements is incorrect. Our bodies have different needs and therefore some individuals may require extra support in the form of supplementation whilst others may get away without taking any supplements. Also, the needs of our bodies may change depending on our stress levels and other lifestyle factors, current diet, as well as our age; and so may our nutritional requirements change accordingly. Due to these changes we may need extra supplementation for only a period of time.

In an ideal world we would get all that we need from the food we eat. Indeed, food should ideally be our medicine. Choosing a wide range of fresh fruits and vegetables of different colours, wholegrains, lean animal products, eggs, beans and other legumes, as well as nuts and seeds, helps to ensure we are getting enough nutrients.

Unfortunately, our diets can be lacking in certain nutrients due to poor nutritional choices, lack of available fresh foods or access to fresh foods, and even due to poor soil quality, which compromises the vitamin and mineral content of the produce we eat.

I encounter a number of common deficiencies in clinical practice including:

- **Zinc** - can lead to brittle hair and nails, poor energy, hair loss, digestive issues and poor wound healing.
- **Iodine** - can lead to thyroid problems resulting in fatigue and weight changes.

- **Iron** - can lead to anaemia and fatigue.
- **Vitamin B12** - can lead to anaemia and fatigue.
- **Magnesium** - can lead to cramping, heart palpitations and constipation.
- **Vitamin D** - can lead to osteoporosis, and may even lead to difficulty losing weight, autoimmune conditions, depression and certain types of cancer.

These deficiencies, luckily, can be detected by laboratory testing and are worth having tested annually.

There are other deficiencies that cannot be laboratory tested. These are vitamins A, B6, C, E, K, and potassium, selenium, as well as antioxidants[1]. Largely these deficiencies are blamed on poor nutritional intake of the foods listed above. As a general rule I do not prescribe these nutrients unless I suspect from someone's lifestyle, diet and/or symptoms that they may be deficient.

Aside from the above common deficiencies there are certain circumstances where supplementation is recommended regardless of laboratory testing.

These include:

- **Folate** - in women planning to conceive and in the first 3 months of pregnancy. Also recommended in the situation of high homocysteine blood levels (a measure of heart attack and stroke risk). Also given to individuals on certain anti-epileptic medications as well as methotrexate medication.
- **B12** - often given in cases of pernicious anaemia by injection.
- **Calcium** - often recommended for postmenopausal women who do not have enough calcium in their diet. It is important to have a magnesium supplement as well as calcium.
- **Coenzyme Q10** - this is important for energy production and is inhibited in those taking a Statin for high cholesterol therefore increasing the risk of muscle soreness. For those taking a Statin it is recommended to take coenzyme Q10 in its active form, ubiquinol, or reduced form to improve absorption into body cells. Some natural medicine practitioners also recommend coenzyme Q10 in those older than 50 years to improve energy as the natural production of coenzyme Q10 reduces with age.
- **Thiamine (vitamin B1)** - often given in the case of alcoholism to prevent brain damage from alcohol poisoning.
- **Vitamin K** - given as either an injection or in its oral form to newborns to prevent potential bleeding due to low vitamin K body stores (vitamin K is used in blood clotting).
- **Omega-3 fatty acids** - often included in infant formula and thought to improve brain

and cellular function. They are often also recommended in those older than 60 years as a blood thinner and anti-inflammatory agent.

- **Vitamin B6** – often given in cases of mild morning sickness as well as for PMS.
- **Multivitamin/multimineral** – given in cases where nutrition is lacking due to poor intake, poor absorption of food nutrients due to certain medical conditions, or due to medical conditions that cause an increase in nutritional requirements. I generally do not recommend multivitamins/multiminerals for everyone as they are not tailored to individual needs.

When Could Taking A Supplement Be Harmful?

There are certain situations when taking a supplement could actually do you harm. This includes taking:

- **Iron** (in those who store too much iron)
- **St John's Wort** (in those on the oral contraceptive pill)
- **Gingko biloba** (in those on blood thinners)
- **Liquorice extract** (in those who have high blood pressure)
- **Copper** (in those who genetically retain copper)
- **Calcium** (in those who have heart disease)
- **Megadoses** (in those taking large doses of supplements for a long period of time, which can actually do more harm than good)

How to Choose Quality Supplements

The production of nutritional supplements has become big business and there is a huge variation in the quality of those sold. To reduce the cost of supplements some companies add various fillers, hydrogenated oils, artificial colours, flavours or sweeteners, or various unwanted excipients. The supplement industry is not tightly regulated or standardised and therefore is largely subject to professional discretion. You cannot always trust that what you are buying is good quality. In essence, you get what you pay for. Do buy your supplements from a reputable source and do spend a little bit more in order to purchase better quality supplements.

Keep in mind that most nutrients work in synergy with other nutrients and not in isolation. So taking high doses of one particular nutrient may cause an imbalance and therefore not have the desired positive effects. The better approach in my opinion would be to see a health-care practitioner trained in the safe and appropriate prescribing of nutritional supplements. For a list of practitioners in Australia and New Zealand refer to the Australasian College of Nutritional and Environmental Medicine (ACNEM) or the Australasian Academy of Anti-Ageing Medicine (A5M).

Take Home Points

There are numerous supplements available for purchase today.

- Not everyone should take supplements and the same supplement does not necessarily suit everyone.
- Ideally, we should be getting all the nutrients we need from the foods we eat.
- Unfortunately our diets can be deficient in nutrients due to poor food choices and reduced soil quality.
- Other situations will increase our requirement for certain nutrients, including during times of stress, chronic infection or illness, pregnancy, or if we are engaging in heavy exercise training, and as we age.
- Some common deficiencies are seen in clinical practice and these can be tested by laboratory testing. They include vitamins D and B12, zinc, iron, iodine, folate and magnesium.
- Other deficiencies include vitamins E, A, C, B6, and K, as well as selenium, potassium and antioxidants. These cannot be accurately laboratory tested and are treated based on symptoms of deficiency.
- In certain situations supplements are used regardless of laboratory testing results, e.g. the use of folate in pregnancy, thiamine in alcoholism, coenzyme Q10 if taking a Statin.
- Other times supplements can be harmful, including taking iron in those who store iron either genetically or as a result of fatty liver disease, taking copper in those who store copper genetically, and taking high doses of fish oil in those already taking blood thinners.
- It is worth consulting with a trained health-care practitioner before taking any supplements to ensure you are taking the correct ones for your body.

YOUR *Weekly* CHALLENGE . . . .

This week your challenge is to stop taking any unnecessary supplements and work on optimising your diet if you have not done so already. If you feel that you may still be lacking in certain nutrients then consider speaking with a healthcare practitioner to have these tested and properly diagnosed.

break addictions

In clinical practice I come across many individuals who struggle with one addiction or another. These can range from addictions to particular substances like tobacco, alcohol, caffeine, illicit drugs, prescription medication and food, to particular activities such as gambling, pornography, shopping, exercise, and even to work. They can be subtle and fairly well disguised by that person and may not impact their lives in general. However every addiction at some point will start to affect a person's physical and mental health, relationships and overall well-being. For this reason, if you are struggling with some sort of addiction and you know it is impacting your life in some way consider trialling some of the suggestions below to break that addiction's stronghold.

Health TIP

One of the most common addictions is alcohol, with the average Australian drinking the equivalent of over 9 L of pure alcohol annually[1].

How to Recognise If You Are Addicted

Determining whether you have an addiction is not as straightforward as you would think. Many a time this is because the addiction is part of your usual routine and behaviour and so has become part of your 'normal'. Also, because admitting you have an addiction is not easy and comes with a social stigma. It can be difficult to want to recognise when this might be the case in your own life. Keep in mind that many people struggle with an addiction of some sort at some stage in their lives and often flip between addictions. However, recovery is not an impossibility.

Consider the questions below. If you answer 'yes' to any of them then you may have an addiction, whether it be to a substance or a particular behaviour.

- Do you regularly or continually use a substance or engage in a certain behaviour as a way to cope emotionally, socially or physically?
- Do you use more of the substance or engage in the behavior more often now than in the past?
- Do you have withdrawal symptoms when you don't have the substance or engage in the behavior?
- Have you lied to anyone about your use of the substance or extent of your behavior?

Recognising when you have an addiction to a substance or a certain behaviour is the first step in being able to break its power in your life.

How Do Addictions Happen?

We become addicted to a substance that we find both pleasurable and rewarding in some way. For an addiction to occur there needs to be a pay-off; at least initially. The area of our brain that is involved in addictions is called the 'Reward Centre' and is a complex circuitry of different brain pathways and brain chemicals, particularly dopamine. When we engage in activities or take substances that trigger the Reward Centre in our brain we experience a 'high' that can be subtle or quite noticeable. Since this emotional experience is a pleasurable one we can become hooked on wanting to engage in that activity and substance again. Some activities and substances are more likely to cause this, particularly nicotine, alcohol and illicit substances due to other chemicals in these substances causing reinforcement of the brains pleasure circuitry.

If we continue to take that particular substance or engage in the activity that we found pleasurable we can establish a neural pathway in our brain such that our brain continually seeks to repeat it. This is much like a train track that we build in our brains that establishes a path of thinking and behaving.

For this reason, current science recognises addiction as a chronic disease that changes both brain structure and function. Just as heart disease damages the heart and diabetes impairs the pancreas, addiction hijacks the brain. This happens as the brain goes through a series of changes, beginning with recognition of pleasure and ending with a drive towards compulsive behaviour even if you no longer want to participate in that behaviour. The end point of addiction is that it seems to take on a life of its own. Luckily, addictions can be broken. Before we look at some of the steps you can take to break an addiction in your life consider whether you may have an addictive personality.

Could You Have an Addictive Personality?

I often get asked whether someone could have an addictive personality. The answer to this question is possibly. Current research suggests that there is not one type of personality that exists that is particularly predisposed to addiction. Saying that, there are factors that can lead someone to addiction, including a combination of certain psychological, social, biological and relational factors.

In clinical practice those individuals I encounter who are more likely to become addicted to a substance or behaviour usually have one or more of the following:

- Suffer from poor self-esteem
- Suffer from anxiety and/or depression
- Have heightened stress and lack coping skills
- Have experienced trauma, especially childhood trauma
- Display a level of impulsivity
- Have a parent or other close family member, partner or someone else in their immediate social circle who is regularly engaged with a particular addictive substance or in a certain behaviour.

So although there is not one addictive personality type per se, if you have developed an addiction to one particular substance or behaviour, then this suggests you have factors underlying your psychology or physiology make-up that make you susceptible to developing other addictions. However, if those factors were identified and dealt with in a healthy way then addictions may be a thing of your past. Let us explore what some of the steps to overcoming addiction might involve.

How to Break an Addiction

STEP 1 – RECOGNISE YOUR 'WHY'

The first step in overcoming an addiction, aside from admitting that you have one, is to do some self-evaluation. Determine why you might be using a substance or engaging in a particular activity. Is it a way for you to cope with stress, anxiety, fatigue, depression or self-loathing? Is it to feel loved, included in a group, or to have fun and experience pleasure? There is always an underlying emotion involved in an addiction so ask yourself what your particular emotion might be.

STEP 2 – CONSIDER ALTERNATIVES

Consider when an addiction is no longer serving you but rather you are serving the addiction. If the underlying reason you have become addicted to a substance has not resolved then you will need to find alternative ways to cope. These ways need to be positive and healthy. In order to break a habit you need to replace it with something else. That 'something else' may be, for example, speaking with a counsellor or good friend, going for a walk, taking up a hobby, buying a pet to love and care for, deep breathing and meditation, or even journaling your thoughts and emotions to get them outside your mind and on paper.

STEP 3 – IDENTIFY YOUR TRIGGER TIMES

A trigger time is a particular time of day, or a situation, that causes you to feel like engaging in your addiction. Recognise when those times might be and do something that is incompatible with your addiction. If your addiction is to drink another glass of wine after dinner as a way to unwind from the stress of your day, consider going for a walk instead, which will force you to get out of the house and not pour another glass.

STEP 4 – SET YOUR LIFE UP FOR SUCCESS

Breaking an addiction is not about willpower, it is about setting yourself up so that you don't succumb to temptation. This might mean, for example, not driving past the bottle shop on the way home but taking an alternate route. Or if pornography is your issue, consider putting the computer in the lounge room in full view of your family. The best way to break an addiction is not to have access to that substance or behaviour.

STEP 5 – BE ACCOUNTABLE

Accountability to someone else will help you stay on track. Consider joining a support group and enlisting the help of your family and friends to help you break an addiction. This of course means admitting to them that you have a problem in the first place. You will be surprised how empowered you feel after taking that step and you will find that addiction will have loosened its hold on you. This is because, deep down, shame is the engine that drives most addictions. As long as you can beat the fear of feeling ashamed and seek help in this area the addiction will soon be a thing of the past.

One patient of mine had a secret addiction to over-the-counter pain medication for many years. She was taking up to 3 times the recommended dose every day as a way to cope with stress. It took her around 12 months to finally admit to me that she had this addiction, but after she did, within a few months she was completely free of using those pain medications. So deep was her level of shame over this secret life that she was living, when she eventually came clean she felt such a sense of relief and empowerment she no longer felt the need to self-medicate.

Overcoming an addiction can be very difficult, but it can be done. When you see yourself making progress, even baby steps, you have to motivate yourself to keep going, so remember to reward yourself along the way (but not with the addictive substance!).

Where to Go If You Need Further Help

If you are really struggling with an addiction in your life then perhaps it may be time to seek help from your health-care professional who is experienced in dealing with addictions and can make the process easier. Keep in mind that breaking an addiction will involve relapse. This is normal and part of the process. The key is to not give up and to try again.

Take Home Points

- Addictions are common and range from being hooked on substances such as alcohol, tobacco, caffeine, food and illicit drugs to certain behaviours such as exercise, shopping, gambling, pornography, and even to work.
- Addictions occur due to activation and reinforcement of the Reward Centre in the brain. This means that as we engage in addictions we develop a neural pathway that essentially etches in our brain that particular behaviour. The result is a compulsion to engage in that behaviour again and again.
- To break the cycle of addiction we can take steps to firstly recognise why we engaged in that addiction, look for alternative coping strategies, identify and avoid our trigger times, become accountable, and reward our efforts along the way.
- Realise that relapse is part of the normal process of breaking an addiction and should be expected. It is not a sign of failure but means that we need to keep going and try again if we are to loosen the grip of our addiction for good.
- Although there is not one particular personality type that is more prone to developing addictions, there are a few factors that can make a person more susceptible to such as lifestyle factors, social factors, and emotional factors. These all need to be individually dealt with to break an addiction in our lives.
- Help for addictions is available and speaking with your health-care professional may be an important first step in breaking an addiction.

YOUR *Weekly* CHALLENGE . . . .

This week your challenge is to identify if you are suffering from an addiction and start making changes to break that addiction in your life. Consider speaking with your health-care professional about this.

cut yourself some slack

Many of us are too hard on ourselves. No more so than in the area of eating habits, lifestyle choices and body weight. Whether it is lamenting over the fact that we no longer fit into those pre-pregnancy jeans, or that we now have areas of our bodies that wobble more than they did last year, or that we lack the willpower of Michelle Bridges, there appears to be a consistent attitude when it comes to how we relate to ourselves. We are our toughest critics.

Health TIP . . . .

Self-criticism can lock us in a state of being unable to change, both mentally and physically. Self-compassion is the key to unlocking this state.

This pattern of thinking creates more harm than good. It can actually work against us to reinforce our negative self-view and worsen confidence and actually perpetuate the behaviour we are trying to avoid. Negative thinking about ourselves can lock us in a state of being unable to change, both physically and emotionally.

Take a patient of mine named Sarah, who came to see me stating that she was unable to lose weight following the birth of her son 5 years ago. She proceeded to point to areas of her body that she disliked most with a look of great disgust. Sarah mentioned that her poor self-image meant that she felt uncomfortable in social situations and refused to be touched by her husband. To try to lose the extra kilos of body weight Sarah had tried 'everything', including expensive weight-loss pills, personal trainers, various diets and had even resorted to dangerously taking too much of her thyroid medication in an attempt to speed up her metabolism.

Although I empathised with Sarah, I suggested that possibly there was another way to help her lose the weight without having to try so hard. I suggested to her that her constant self-denigration had created a state of anxiety and stress in her body. This state in turn had increased stress hormone levels. Stress hormones act as a diabetic agent – they increase blood sugar levels, prevent weight loss, cause abdominal weight gain, in particular, and lower metabolism. Her body was fighting her best efforts to lose weight. Her body was doing what it was programmed to do – survive – and therefore store body fat. To reverse this process Sarah would have to learn to live in a state of reduced stress levels and the first step in doing so was to extend to herself a little compassion. Self-compassion is key to long-term positive change.

What Exactly Is Self-Compassion?

Self-compassion is a relatively new term in psychology circles and essentially refers to cutting yourself some slack. As Dr Kristin Neff, Associate Professor in Human Development and Culture at the University of Texas, put it in her latest TedX talk, '…Instead of mercilessly judging and criticising yourself for various inadequacies or shortcomings, self-compassion means you are kind and understanding when confronted with personal failings – after all, who ever said you were supposed to be perfect? You may try to change in ways that allow you to be more healthy and happy, but this is done because you care about yourself, not because you are worthless or unacceptable [1].'

There will be situations in our lives that we dislike and even frustrate us. This is a common human experience. But by extending a little grace to ourselves we can learn to continue to move forward without getting stuck in a vicious cycle of shame and self-defeating behaviour.

When I mentioned this to Sarah, she seemed opposed initially to the idea of self-compassion. She was afraid that if she loosened the reins on herself she would, in her own terms, '… get even fatter'. But after a little convincing she was courageous enough, and perhaps so frustrated at her previous attempts, that she decided to give it a try. By reducing her need to strive for perfection with regards to her eating habits Sarah noticed that she was no longer succumbing to binge eating. She was able to make better choices with regards to her eating without getting stuck in the cycle of deprivation. By reducing her need to strive for perfection with regards to exercise she no longer felt the need to train for 2 hours every day. This reduction in excessive activity not only reduced the stress levels in her body but she found that she had extra time to spend with her husband and son. Overall, after just a few short months Sarah was a much happier and healthier person. She had stopped focussing on her body weight as a measure of self-worth and had started to focus on other much more important aspects of her life; namely her relationship with herself and her significant others.

Sarah's story highlights how important self-compassion is in the process of making positive lifestyle and health changes. However, before you can extend to yourself some compassion it is important to understand what distinguishes self-compassion from other areas of positive psychology.

What Self-Compassion Is Not

Self-compassion is a distinct concept and should not to be confused with the following similar but subtly different terms:

Self-pity When individuals feel self-pity they become immersed in their own problems and forget that others have similar problems. This can make them self-absorbed, and introspective. Self-compassion, on-the-other-hand, says that as humans we all have shared common experiences, including suffering, and there is always someone else worse off.

Self-indulgence Being compassionate to oneself does not mean you allow yourself to get away with everything, especially harmful behaviours. A central premise of self-compassion is that you want to be happy and healthy in the long-term, even if this means feeling a little discomfort in the meantime.

Self-esteem To some degree self-esteem relies on external cues that you are okay such as others commenting on your looks or behaviour. Therefore self-esteem is based on comparison with others and whether you feel you deserve to feel good about yourself. Self-compassion on the other hand says that you deserve compassion because all human beings deserve compassion and understanding. This means that with self-compassion you do not have to feel better than others to feel good about yourself.

Health TIP

Consider treating yourself as your own best friend. After all, we teach people how to treat us and if we treat ourselves badly others will have permission to do the same.

How to Practise Self-Compassion

To get the idea of what self-compassion would look like in your own life try the following exercise[2]. Take out a piece of paper and write down answers to the following questions.

1 Think about a time when a close friend was feeling really bad about themselves or their behaviour. Consider how you responded or would respond to them in this

situation. Write down what you typically do, what you say, and note the tone in which you typically talk to your friends.

2 Now think about a recent time when you felt bad about yourself. How do you typically respond to *yourself* in these situations? Please write down what you typically do, what you say, and note the tone in which you talk to yourself.

3 Did you notice a difference? If so, ask yourself why. Are there any factors or influences that come into play that lead you to treat yourself and others so differently?

4 Please write down how you think things might change if you responded to yourself in the same way you typically respond to a close friend when you are suffering. Would you feel more energised to want to move forward, would you feel more positive about your future and your outlook, would you be more self-accepting?

Take Home Points

Self-compassion means cutting yourself some slack every now and then.

- When we are locked in a vicious cycle of shame, guilt and self-hatred we can become paralysed and unable to change our behaviours. In this state our bodies will fight our best efforts to make positive changes.

- The key to self-compassion is to extend to yourself the same grace you would to a close friend when they are feeling down about themselves.

- This attitude of acceptance rather than self-denigration helps our bodies and minds to move forward to a more positive way of living.

- Self-compassion should not, however, be confused with self-pity, self-indulgence or self-esteem, which are distinct concepts.

- Self-compassion is not a default emotion that many of us feel towards ourselves but rather a learnt skill.

YOUR *Weekly* CHALLENGE . . . .

This week your challenge is to practise self-compassion. For situations where you would normally beat yourself up about missing the mark consider extending to yourself a little grace, not as an excuse to continue harmful behaviours but rather as recognition that you are not going be able to behave perfectly all the time.

putting your prescription into practice

So now that you have reached the end of *Healthy Habits* you are well and truly familiar with what you need to do to improve your health for the long-term. Perhaps you followed this book from start to finish and 12 months have now passed. Hopefully you have been tracking your progress and are happy with your positive changes and results. But if you have found it difficult to stay on track then go back and revise the summary sections of each chapter. Perhaps commit to another 12 months to consolidate your positive habits. Some other strategies for putting 'your prescription' of good habits into practice include:

- **Strengthen Your Why** Determine why is it you want to change. The stronger your 'why' the more likely you are not to give up. Write out all the pros and cons of staying the same versus changing. This might just help to keep you focussed.

- **Focus on Emotion** Emotions are powerful things. We often make decisions not based on reason but on emotion. If you are finding it difficult to stay on track with positive changes try to associate that positive change with how you will feel if you achieve that change e.g. more energetic, more attractive, more vibrant, and/or happier and more confident.

- **Be Consistent** Cractice is the key to establishing positive habits. Try and be as consistent as you can and soon enough you will find that you have created a new, effortless habit.

- **Be Patient** Change takes time. Nothing worth achieving happens overnight. Give yourself time to change and rest knowing that each day you are implementing a positive habit is another day moving towards your goal.

- **Keep the End Goal in Sight** Sometimes it is hard to persist with positive changes if the end is not in sight. Focussing on the end goal often helps to keep us focussed. Consider sticking your goal tracker on the refrigerator door. That way you are reminded of the end goal, that is, achieving a year of implementing positive changes.

- **Create Accountability** Along with keeping your end goal in sight, remember to establish accountability. This was mentioned at the start of this book but can not be emphasised enough. Accountability to someone else often means you will keep going when you ordinarily would have given up. Consider asking a close friend, family member or doctor to keep you accountable to your progress with the 52 Simple Habits.

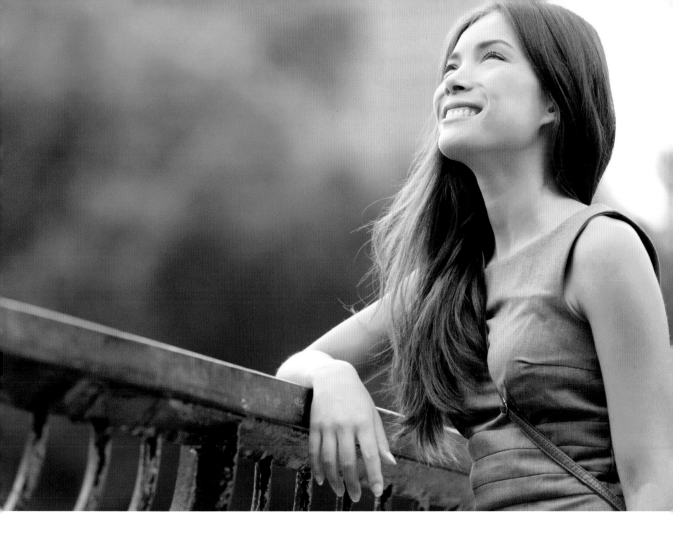

Give them permission to ask you regularly how you are going with implementing them into your lifestyle.

- **Choose Your Time Wisely** Sometimes we try to change our lifestyles and it is not the best time to do so. Recognise when life is not stable enough to provide time and emotional space to make positive changes. Come back to making positive changes later when things have settled down. Set a date to revisit making the positive changes in this book, though, otherwise you might procrastinate indefinitely.

- **Create Rewards** To keep yourself motivated consider creating rewards (non-food based!) along the way. Perhaps for every 5 or so habits you introduce into your lifestyle consider celebrating by enjoying a day out with friends or family or buying yourself a little gift as a token to remind you of what you have achieved.

Now that you have filled your prescription to great health, allow me to take my doctor coat off, so to speak, and give you a big hug as a friend, for a job well done. You should be proud of your changes!

a final word

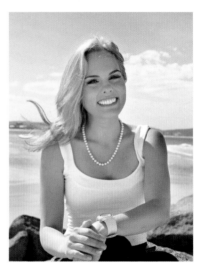

To leave you with a final thought, consider that all of life is merely an experience and a journey. That journey will be marked by struggles and triumphs, joys and sadness, highs and lows, and moving forwards and sometimes backwards. In order to experience that journey to the fullest, with all of its ups and downs, we need to be as healthy as we can. Consider that one of our most valuable assets is our health. It is something that no one can gain for you; no amount of money can buy back for you once it is lost; and very little compares to the satisfaction of working towards attaining it.

It is easy to think that once you have 'perfect' health you will be fulfilled but it is actually the working towards attaining good health, much like any other goal, that is the most rewarding part of the journey. Remember that through your endeavour to make positive changes, however difficult they might feel initially, you will receive the reward of reaching your goal. This creates a sense of confidence and personal self-mastery. Little by little, change by change, your lifestyle is transformed, and with it your health and your experience of life. Remember to keep focussed, be consistent, stay positive, and praise your efforts. Your reward of great health and a waistline to match is within reach and yours for the keeping.

your 52 simple habits prescription

Use the following two pages of tables as your week-by-week 'Simple Habits Prescription'. Consider photocopying each page and sticking it on your refrigerator or bathroom mirror as a way to visually track your progress. Each table is divided into 26 weeks or 6 months of the sequential habits presented in this book. Place a tick next to the week and habit once you have completed that chapter but also have attempted to incorporate that habit into your lifestyle. If you have already previously mastered that habit before even reading this book, go ahead and tick it at the start of the week and continue to work on the other habits. As you progress through the reading of this book as a way of remembering the other habits continue to tick them at the appropriate week to track their ongoing incorporation into your lifestyle.

Habit	1	2	3	4	5	6	7	8	9	10	11	12	13	14	15	16	17	18	19	20	21	22	23	24	25	26
know your motivators																										
drink to good health																										
avoid shrinking your brain																										
sleep well																										
rest & recover																										
restore your biorhythms																										
eat by the 80/20 rule																										
clean out your pantry																										
pack a healthy lunchbox																										
balance your blood sugar																										
eat a rainbow a day																										
eat with the seasons																										
eat out with confidence																										
buy smart & don't spend a fortune																										
plan well, plan to succeed																										
practice portion perfection																										
reduce mindless eating																										
listen to your hunger cues																										
overcome cravings																										
say die to dieting forever																										
be healthy at any size																										
stay regular																										
digest well																										
recognise food upsets																										
detox & love your liver																										
say goodbye to toxic stress																										

Habit	WEEK																										
	27	28	29	30	31	32	33	34	35	36	37	38	39	40	41	42	43	44	45	46	47	48	49	50	51	52
avoid overstimulation																										
learn to breathe																										
break negative thought patterns																										
nurture yourself																										
have a health check																										
move more																										
avoid injury																										
look after your posture																										
protect your pelvic floor																										
strengthen your core																										
recognise overtraining																										
boost your metabolism																										
boost your immunity																										
balance your sex hormones																										
boost your happy hormones																										
boost brain alpha waves																										
boost oxytocin, the bonding hormone																										
practise the art of letting go																										
laugh more																										
recognise allergies																										
get some sunshine																										
love the skin you are in																										
ward off cancer cells																										
choose supplements wisely																										
break addictions																										
cut yourself some slack																										

a closer look at common fad diets

DIET	DESCRIPTION
Paleo Diet	This diet essentially excludes all grains and starchy vegetables. Its premise is that we should live as we did as cave men and women and not eat any processed food. It is high in protein, non-starchy vegetables and salads and low in natural fructose sugar. The issue with this diet is that it excludes grains, which may prove unsustainable. Also, wholegrains have been found to lower the risk of bowel cancer and so excluding these from the diet may put individuals at risk.
Alkaline Diet	This diet involves consuming only foods that are supposed to increase the alkalinity of the tissues and reduce acidity. Acidity has been attributed to development of chronic disease, cancer and joint pains. Acidic foods include dairy, eggs, meats, grains, and some fruits and vegetables. The issue comes when individuals exclude major food groups in an attempt to stay as 'alkaline' as possible. Moderation is the key as it is now thought that perhaps it is the quantity and unbalanced amount of acidic foods over alkaline foods that actually is the cause of illness and not the individual foods per se.
High-Protein Diet	This diet involves eating very high amounts of protein to the exclusion of carbohydrates. Although this diet will result in weight loss, it is high in saturated fat, can reduce physical and mental performance, is not sustainable, and can cause kidney damage. This diet is not recommended. A healthy eating plan includes balanced amounts of protein and carbohydrates in a portion-controlled manner to ensure no major food group is omitted and health is not put at risk.
Low-Carb Diet	See above for high-protein diet
No-Sugar Diet	This diet involves removing all sugar from the diet including fructose sugar found in fruits, some starchy vegetables and honey. It is thought that by removing sugar from the diet insulin spikes do not occur and the liver cannot therefore convert sugar into fat. This diet too can prove unsustainable and by omitting fruit altogether you can develop constipation and have reduced vitamin and mineral intake. A more balanced approach would be to reduce processed and hidden sugars which are thought to contribute to the major issue of weight gain in today's society.

DIET	DESCRIPTION
Juice-Only Diet	This diet claims that by drinking just fresh fruit juice and/or vegetable juice for a set period of time weight will be lost and toxins removed from the body. Although this may be true, this type of diet is not healthy or sustainable. It can lead to blood sugar problems, muscle mass loss and lack of energy.
Fasting	This diet claims that by completely avoiding food and drinks other than water for a set period of time then weight will be lost and toxins removed from the body. Although this may be true, once again this type of diet is not sustainable and may be harmful for certain individuals especially for those with some chronic health conditions like diabetes. It is not recommended as part of a healthy eating plan and risks creating a vicious cycle of binge-eating and yo-yo dieting.
HCG Diet	This diet is based on a 500 Calorie diet for 3 weeks in conjunction with taking a medication that is pregnancy hormone (human chorionic gonadotropin (hCG)). It results in rapid weight loss. The problem with this diet is that if an individual has not changed their lifestyle when coming off the diet then there is the risk of putting the weight back on. Also, restricting Calories to this low level can result in gallstone formation in some individuals. The absolute safety of taking hCG is yet to be definitely proven in studies.
Blood-Type Diet	This diet involves eating only certain foods that are approved for your blood type. It involves strict adherence to food rules and can be restrictive. It is not recommended as it has not been proven to be beneficial and may result in nutrient deficiencies.
Body Type Diet	This diet involves eating only certain types of foods and avoiding others that may not agree with your body type. It has not been proven to be effective in causing greater weight loss or health benefits over other types of healthy eating plans.
Atkins Diet	See above for high-protein diet
Raw Food Diet	This diet involves eating only raw foods and does not permit foods to be cooked. The premise here being that cooking destroys natural enzymes and nutrients in foods. Although there is nothing essentially wrong with this diet it is not sustainable and can omit food groups in an attempt to include raw foods only.
Shake Diet	This diet involves replacing one or more meals with a low-calorie protein shake. Although this diet will result in weight loss it has found not to be sustainable in the long-term and can quickly result in regaining lost weight once normal eating resumes.

food additives to avoid

Below is a list of food additives and their respective codes to avoid if you have or suspect chemical sensitivities. Feel free to photocopy this list or take a photo of it with your mobile so that you can take it along with you when you food shop.

COLOURS	
Artificial	102, 107, 110, 122-129, 132, 133, 142, 151, 155
Natural	160B (annatto)
PRESERVATIVES	
Sorbates	200-203
Benzoates	210-218
Sulphites	220-228
Nitrates, Nitrites	249-252
Proprionates	280-283
Antioxidants	310-312, 319-321
FLAVOUR ENHANCERS	
Glutamate (e.g. MSG)	621-635
Hydrolysed Vegetable Protein	HVP
Textured Vegetable Protein	TVP

references

1 Habit Formation: The Key to Getting & Staying Healthy is Found in Your Habits
2 Sentence comprehension: The integration of habits and rules. David J. Townsend and Thomas G. Bever. Cambridge, MA: MIT Press, 2001. Pp. 455

Simple Health Habit #1 – Know Your Motivators

1 World Health Organisation. 2003. Adherence to Long-Term Therapies: Evidence for action. http://apps.who.int/medicinedocs/en/d/Js4883e/5.html (accessed Jan 2015).
2 Prochaska, J and Diclemente, C. Treating Addictive Behaviours: Processes of change. 1986. Springer, USA.

Simple Health Habit #2 – Drink To Good Health

1 The USGS Water Science School, "What Does Water do for You", http://www.ga.water.usgs.gov/edu/propertyyou.html (accessed January 20th 2014).
2 Live Science, "How Long Can a Person Survive without Water", http://www.livescience.com/32320-how-long-can-a-person-survive-without-water.html (accessed January 20th 2014).
3 Mayo Clinic, Symptoms of Dehydration, http://www.mayoclinic.org/diseases-conditions/dehydration/basics/symptoms/con-20030056 (accessed January 20th 2014).
4 Colbert, D M.D. 2007, The Seven Pillars of Health, Siloam Publishing, Florida.
5 Better Health Channel, "Muscle Cramp", http://www.betterhealth.vic.gov.au/bhcv2/bhcarticles.nsf/pages/Muscle_cramp (accessed January 20th 2014).
6 Better Health Channel, "Water – a vital nutrient", http://www.betterhealth.vic.gov.au/bhcv2/bhcarticles.nsf/pages/Water_a_vital_nutrient (accessed January 20th 2014).
7 Australian Institute of Sport, "Fluid – who needs it?" http://www.ausport.gov.au/ais/nutrition/factsheets/hydration/fluid_-_who_needs_it (accessed January 21st 2014).
8 Mayo Clinic, "Dehydration treatment and drugs, http://www.mayoclinic.org/diseases-conditions/dehydration/basics/treatment/con-20030056 (accessed January 21st 2014).
9 Better Health Channel, "Water – tanks, bores and dams", http://www.betterhealth.vic.gov.au/bhcv2/bhcarticles.nsf/pages/Water_tanks_bores_and_dams?open (accessed January 21st 2014).

Simple Health Habit #3 – Avoid Shrinking Your Brain

1 The USGS Water Science School, "The water in you", http://www.ga.water.usgs.gov/edu/propertyyou.html (accessed July 2014).
2 Live Science, "How Long Can a Person Survive without Water", http://www.livescience.com/32320-how-long-can-a-person-survive-without-water.html (accessed January 20th 2014).
3 Mayo Clinic, Symptoms of Dehydration, http://www.mayoclinic.org/diseases-conditions/dehydration/basics/symptoms/con-20030056 (accessed January 20th 2014).
4 Kempton MJ et al 2011. Dehydration affects brain structure and function in healthy adolescents. Hum Brain Mapp. Jan;32(1):71-9.
5 Australian Drug Foundation, "Caffeine facts", http://www.druginfo.adf.org.au/drug-facts/caffeine (accessed July 2014).

6 Australian Beverages, "Caffeine – the facts", http://australianbeverages.org/for-consumers/caffeine-facts/ (accessed July 2014).
7 National Institute on Alcohol Abuse and Alcoholism, "Alcohol Alert", http://pubs.niaaa.nih.gov/publications/aa63/aa63.htm (accessed July 2014).
8 Australian Government Department of Health, "Alcohol – reduce your risk", http://www.alcohol.gov.au/internet/alcohol/publishing.nsf/Content/guide-adult (accessed July 2014)

Simple Health Habit #4 – Sleep Well

1 The Medical Journal of Australia, 2013. Insomnia: prevalence, consequences, and effective treatment. https://www.mja.com.au/journal/2013/199/8/insomnia-prevalence-consequences-and-effective-treatment (accessed Aug 2014).
2 American Psychological Association 2005, Sleep. http://www.apa.org/topics/sleep/why.aspx?item=4 (accessed Aug 2014).
3 Harvard Medical School 2006. Importance of Sleep http://www.health.harvard.edu/press_releases/importance_of_sleep_and_health (accessed Aug 2014).
4 Sleep Health Foundation 2013. Sleep Health Facts http://www.sleephealthfoundation.org.au/tip-of-the-week/331-an-hour-before-midnight-is-worth-two-after.html (accessed Aug 2014)
5 The National Sleep Research Project, 2000. 40 Amazing Facts About Sleep. http://www.abc.net.au/science/sleep/facts.htm (accessed Aug 2014)

Simple Health Habit #5 – Rest & Recover

1 Psychology Today. 2012. Where do you fall on the burn-out continuum. http://www.psychologytoday.com/blog/high-octane-women/201205/where-do-you-fall-the-burnout-continuum (accessed Aug 2014).
2 Polyphasic Society 2014. Basic Rest & Activity Cycles. https://www.washington.edu/admin/hr/benefits/publications/carelink/tipsheets/rest-relax.pdf (accessed Aug 2014).
3 Black Dog Institute 2014. Mindfulness in Everyday Life. http://www.blackdoginstitute.org.au/docs/10.mindfulnessineverydaylife.pdf (accessed Aug 2014).
4 Scientific American 2013. Why Your Brain Needs More Downtime. http://www.scientificamerican.com/article/mental-downtime/ (accessed Aug 2014).

Simple Health Habit #9 – Pack Your Lunchbox Wisely

1 Colbert, D. M.D. Eat This and Live. Siloam. 2009. Florida, USA.

Simple Health Habit #10 – Balance Your Blood Sugar

1 Diabetes Australia. 2013. Diabetes in Australia. http://www.diabetesaustralia.com.au/Understanding-Diabetes/Diabetes-in-Australia/ (accessed Dec 2014).

Simple Health Habit #11 – Eat a Rainbow A Day

1 Gupta C, Prakash D. 2014. Phytonutrients as therapeutic agents. J Complement Integr Med. 2014 Sep;11(3):151-69.

2 Giovannucci, E. et al. 1995. Intake of carotenoids and retinol in relation to risk of prostate cancer. J Nat Ca Inst. 1995; 87: 1767-1776

3 NYU Langone Medical Centre. 2014. Citrus Bioflavanoids. http://www.med.nyu.edu/content?ChunkIID=21574 (accessed Jan 2015).

4 Franz, M. 2011. Your Brain on Blueberries: Enhance Memory with the Right Foods. Scientific American. Jan/Feb Ed 2011.

5 Seddon, J.M. et al. 1994. Dietary Carotenoids, Vitamins A, C, and E, and Advanced Age-Related Macular Degeneration. JAMA. 1994; 272; 1413-1420.

6 Tilton, S. PhD. 2006. Benefits and Risks of Supplementation with Indole Phytochemicals. Linus Pauling Institute, Oregon State University. http://lpi.oregonstate.edu/ss06/indole.html (accessed Jan 2015).

Simple Health Habit #12 – Eat With the Seasons

1 Greening Princeton Farmers Market, Princeton University https://webscript.princeton.edu/~greening/market/?page_id=58

2 Sustainable Table http://www.sustainabletable.org.au

3 Dr. Decuypere's Nutrient Charts http://www.healthalternatives2000.com/vegetables-nutrition-chart.html

4 Life Organic Seasonal Produce Tables http://www.lifeorganic.com.au/seasonal.htm l

5 The Better Health Channel http://www.betterhealth.vic.gov.au/bhcv2/bhcrecipes.nsf/InSeasonView/InSeason?OpenDocument

6 Organic Trade Association http://www.ota.com/organic/benefits/nutrition.html

Simple Health Habit #13 – Eat Out With Confidence

1 Don Colbert. The Seven Pillars of Health. 2007, Siloam Publishing, USA.

Simple Health Habit #14 – Buy Smart & Don't Spend a Fortune

1 BMJ, 2013. Do healthier foods and diet patterns cost more than less healthy options? A systematic review and meta-analysis. http://bmjopen.bmj.com/content/3/12/e004277.full (Accessed Feb 2014)

2 NHMRC ,2012. Obesity and Overweight. http://www.nhmrc.gov.au/your-health/obesity-and-overweight (Accessed Feb 2014)

3 Preventative Health Task Force, 2005. Obesity. http://www.preventativehealth.org.au/internet/preventativehealth/publishing.nsf/Content/E233F8695823F16CCA2574DD00818E64/$File/obesity-2.pdf (Accessed Feb 2014).

4 MJA, 2013. Cost of Overweight and Obesity in Australia. https://www.mja.com.au/journal/2010/192/5/cost-overweight-and-obesity-australia (Accessed Feb 2014)

5 Business Pundit, 2010. The Cost of Living: Healthhy vs Unhealthy. http://www.businesspundit.com/the-cost-of-living-healthy-vs-unhealthy/ (Accessed Feb 2014)

Simple Health Habit #16 – Practise Portion Perfection

1 Eat for Health. 2013. How Much Do We Need Each Day. https://www.eatforhealth.gov.au/food-essentials/how-much-do-we-need-each-day (accessed Jan 2015).

2 National Health & Medical Research Council. 2013. Eat for Health: Australian Dietary Guidelines. http://www.eatforhealth.gov.au/sites/default/files/files/the_guidelines/n55_australian_dietary_guidelines.pdf (accessed Jan 2015).

3 Wansink, B. Mindless Eating: Why we eat more than we think, 2006, Hay House Australia Ltd, NSW, Australia.

Simple Health Habit #17 – Reduce Mindless Eating

1 Wansink, B. Mindless Eating: Why we eat more than we think, 2006, Hay House Australia Ltd, NSW, Australia.

Simple Health Habit #19 – Overcome Cravings

1 Nishizawa, S. et al. Differences between males and females in rates of serotonin synthesis in human bran. Proceedings of the National Academy of Sciences USA 94 (1997): 5308-5313.

Simple Health Habit #20 – Say Die to Dieting Forever

1 Franz, M. The Answer to Weight Loss is Easy – Doing It Is Hard. Clinical Diabetes. July 2001 vol. 19 no. 3 105-109.

2 Blair-Wes, G. Weight Loss for Food Lovers 3rd Edition: Understanding our minds and why we sabotage our weight loss. 2006. Alclare Pty Ltd, Indooroopilly, Australia.

Simple Health Habit #21 – Be Healthy at Any Size

1 Bacon, L. Health at Every Size. 2008. BenBella Books, Dallas, USA.

Simple Health Habit #22 – Stay Regular

1 National Continence Management Strategy. 2003. Best practice in the prevention and treatment of constipation in adults under 65 years. http://www.health.gov.au/internet/main/publishing.nsf/content/continence-ncms-faecalmgmt.htm/$file/pjt23clinical.pdf (accessed Aug 2014).

2 Heaton, K W & Lewis, S J 1997, 'Stool form scale as a useful guide to intestinal transit time'. *Scandinavian Journal of Gastroenterology*, vol.32, no.9, pp.920 - 924.

3 World Gastroenterology Organisation. 2007. Diverticular Disease. http://www.worldgastroenterology.org/assets/downloads/en/pdf/guidelines/07_diverticular_disease.pdf (accessed Aug 2014).

4 Continence Foundation of Australia. 2014. Faecal Incontinence. http://www.continence.org.au/pages/what-is-incontinence.html (accessed Aug 2014).

5 Science Daily. 2012. Chronic Constipation Linked to Increased Risk of Colorectal Cancer. http://www.sciencedaily.com/releases/2012/10/121022081228.htm (accessed Aug 2014).

Simple Health Habit #23 – Digest Well

1 Mercola. 2012. How Your Gut Flora Influences Your Health. http://articles.mercola.com/sites/articles/archive/2012/06/27/probiotics-gut-health-impact.aspx (accessed Aug 2014).

2 Monash University. 2010. Low FODMAP Diet. http://www.med.monash.edu/cecs/gastro/fodmap/low-high.html (accessed Aug 2014).

3 Rösch W, Vinson B, Sassin I. 2002. A randomised clinical trial comparing the efficacy of a herbal preparation STW 5 with the prokinetic drug cisapride in patients with dysmotility type of functional dyspepsia. Z Gastroenterol. Jun;40(6):401-8.

Simple Health Habit #24 – Recognise Food Upsets

1 Better Health Channel. 2014. Food Allergy & Intolerance. http://www.betterhealth.vic.gov.au/bhcv2/bhcarticles.nsf/pages/food_allergy_and_intolerance (accessed Jan 2015).

2 NSW Food Authority. 2014. Allergy & Intolerance. http://www.foodauthority.nsw.gov.au/consumers/problems-with-food/allergy-and-intolerance#.VK4a6pp-_mQ (accessed Jan 2015).

Simple Health Habit #25 – Detox & Love Your Liver

1 Better Health Chanel. 2011. The Liver. http://www.betterhealth.vic.gov.au/bhcv2/bhcarticles.nsf/pages/Liver_explained (accessed Aug 2014).

2   Pelagria Research Library. 2011. Hepatoprotective effects from the leaf extracts of Brassica juncea in CCl4 induced rat model. http://pelagiaresearchlibrary.com/der-pharmacia-sinica/vol2-iss4/DPS-2011-2-4-274-285.pdf (accessed Aug 2014).

3   M.F. Ahmed et al. 2012. Int. Res. J. of Pharmaceuticals. Protective Effect of Brassica oleracea L. var. capitata against Simvastatin Induced Hepatotoxicity in Rats http://www.scientific-journals.co.uk/web_documents/1020412_brassica_oleracea_protection.pdf (accessed Aug 2014).

4   University of Maryland Medical Center 2014. Milk Thistle. http://umm.edu/health/medical-reference-guide/complementary-and-alternative-medicine-guide/herb/milk-thistle (accessed Aug 2014).

Simple Health Habit #26 - Say Goodbye to Toxic Stress

1   The Department of Health 2014. General Practice Statistics. http://www.health.gov.au/internet/main/publishing.nsf/Content/General +Practice+Statistics-1 (accessed June 2014)

2   American Psychological Association 2014. Stress effects on the body. http://www.apa.org/helpcenter/stress-body.aspx (accessed June 2014)

3   The American Institute of Stress 2014. 50 Common signs and symptoms of stress. http://www.stress.org/stress-effects/ (accessed June 2014)

Simple Health Habit #28 - Learn to Breathe

1   Harvard Health Publications. 2009. Take a deep breath. http://www.health.harvard.edu/newsletters/Harvard_Mental_Health_Letter/2009/May/Take-a-deep-breath (accessed Sep 2014).

Simple Health Habit #29 - Break Negative Thought Patterns

1   Leaf, Caroline. 2009. Who Switched Off My Brain: Controlling toxic thoughts and emotions. Thomas Nelson Publishers, USA.

2   Monash University. 2014. Counselling & Mental Health: Changing Negative Thoughts. http://www.monash.edu.au/counselling/self-help/changing-negative-thoughts.html (accessed Jan 2015).

Simple Health Habit #30 - Nurture Yourself

1   Meyers Gantman, S. 2015. Ways to Nurture Yourself. http://www.straightfromtheheart.com/growth_selfnurture.htm (accessed Jan 2015).

Simple Health Habit #31 - Have a Health Check

1   Australian Institute of Health & Welfare. 2013. Cancer Screening Programs in Australia. http://www.aihw.gov.au/cancer/screening/ (accessed September 2013). s

2   Australian Institute of Health & Welfare. 2013. Bowel Screen. http://www.aihw.gov.au/cancer/screening/bowel/ (accessed September 2013).

Simple Health Habit #32 - Move More

1   Australian Bureau of Statistics. 2013. Exercise. http://www.abs.gov.au/ausstats/abs@.nsf/Lookup/4338.0main+features112011-13 (accessed Jan 2015).

2   Australian Government Department of Health. 2013. Physical Inactivity Facts & Figures. http://www.health.gov.au/internet/main/publishing.nsf/Content/health-pubhlth-strateg-active-evidence.htm (accessed Jan 2015).

3   Better Health Channel. 2014. Physical Activity - It's Important. http://www.betterhealth.vic.gov.au/bhcv2/bhcarticles.nsf/pages/physical_activity_its_important?open (accessed Jan 2015).

4   National Cancer Institute. 2009. Physical Activity and Cancer. http://www.cancer.gov/cancertopics/factsheet/prevention/physicalactivity (accessed Jan 2015).

5   Schilke, J. 1991. Slowing the ageing process with physical activity. J Gerontol Nurs. Jun;17(6):4-8.

Simple Health Habit #33 - Avoid Injury

1   Beer, B. 2015. You Can Run Pain Free: A Physio's 5 Step Guide to Enjoying Injury-Free and Faster Running. Michael Hanrahan Publishing. Victoria, Australia.

Simple Health Habit #35 - Protect Your Pelvic Floor

1   Continence Foundation of Australia. 2006. Key Statistics. http://www.continence.org.au/pages/key-statistics.html (accessed Jan 2015).

Simple Health Habit #36 - Strengthen Your Core

1   Phillips, E. 2012. Harvard Health Publications: Build Your Core Muscles for a Healthier, More Active Future. http://www.health.harvard.edu/blog/build-your-core-muscles-for-a-healthier-more-active-future-201212285698 (accessed Jan 2015).

Simple Health Habit #37 - Recognise Overtraining

1   Elizabeth Quinn. The Benefits of Rest and Recover After Exericse. http://sportsmedicine.about.com/od/sampleworkouts/a/RestandRecovery.htm (accessed Nov 2014)

2   Elizabeth Quinn. Overtraining Syndrome and Athletes. http://sportsmedicine.about.com/cs/overtraining/a/aa062499a.htm (accessed Nov 2014)

3   Uusitalo, A.L.T., Tahvanainen, K.U.O., Uusitalo, A.J., Rusko, H.K.: Does increase in training intensity vs. volume influence supine and standing heart rate and heart rate variability. Overtraining and Overreaching in Sport - Congress, Memphis, Tennessee, 1996.

4   Lamberg, L., Sleep May Be Athletes' Best Performance Booster, Psychiatric News August 19, 2005, Volume 40 Number 16

Simple Health Habit #39 - Boost Your Immunity

1   Science Daily. 2014. Upper Respiratory Tract Infection. http://www.sciencedaily.com/articles/u/upper_respiratory_tract_infection.htm (accessed Jan 2015).

2   Kotsirilos, V et al. A Guide to evidence-based integrative and complementary medicine. 2011. Elsevier Australia.

3   Phelps, K and Hassad, C. General Practice The Integrative Approach. 2011. Elsevier Australia.

4   Sanchez, A. et al. 1973. Role of sugars in human neutrophilic phagocytosis. Am J Clin. vol. 26 no. 11 1180-1184.

Simple Health Habit #40 - Balance Your Sex Hormones

1   Turner, N. The Hormone Diet. Random House Canada. 2009.

Simple Health Habit #41 - Boost Your Happy Hormones

1   Black Dog Institute. 2012 Facts and Figures about Mental Health & Mood Disorders. http://www.blackdoginstitute.org.au/docs/Factsandfiguresaboutmentalhealthandmooddisorders.pdf (accessed Dec 2014)

2   American Psychiatric Association. 2014. Criteria for Major Depressive Episode: DSM 5. http://www.nami.org/Content/NavigationMenu/Intranet/Homefront/Criteria_Major_D_Episode.pdf (accessed Dec 2014).

3   WebMD 2014. Anxiety and Panic Disorders Health Center. http://www.webmd.com/anxiety-panic/guide/mental-health-anxiety-disorders (accessed Dec 2014).

4 Cowen, P.J. Cortisol, serotonin and depression: all stressed out? The British Journal of Psychiatry (2002) 180: 99-100

5 Winston, A.P. et al. Neuropsychiatric effects of caffeine. Advances in Psychiatric Treatment (2005) 11: 432-439.

6 Beyond Blue. 2014. What causes depression? http://www.beyondblue.org.au/the-facts/depression/what-causes-depression (accessed Dec 2014).

7 Better Health Channel. 2012. Exercise and depression. http://www.betterhealth.vic.gov.au/bhcv2/bhcarticles.nsf/pages/Depression_and_exercise (accessed Dec 2014).

Simple Health Habit #42 - Boost Brain Alpha Waves

1 Livestrong. 2011. Exercises to Achieve Alpha Brain Waves. http://www.livestrong.com/article/438650-exercises-to-achieve-alpha-brain-waves/ (accessed Jan 2015).

2 American Psychological Association. 2012. What are the benefits of mindfulness. http://www.apa.org/monitor/2012/07-08/ce-corner.aspx (accessed Jan 2015).

3 Hassed, C. 2012. Mindfulness at Monash: the health benefits of meditation and being mindful. http://www.49.com.au/wp-content/uploads/The-health-benefits-of-meditation-and-being-mindful_v21-2.pdf (accessed Jan 2015).

Simple Health Habit #43 - Boost Oxytocin, the Bonding Hormone

1 Social Connection and Health, Vic Health http://www.vichealth.vic.gov.au/Programs-and-Projects/Social-Connection/Social-connection-and-health-overview.aspx

2 Zak, Paul. 2013. Psychology Today: The Moral Molecule. http://www.psychologytoday.com/blog/the-moral-molecule/201311/the-top-10-ways-boost-good-feelings (accessed Dec 2014)

3 Social Connectedness, Monash University http://www.med.monash.edu.au/sphc/pcru/chrg/av-charge-review.pdf

4 Social Connectedness and Health, Wilder Research http://www.bcbsmnfoundation.org/system/asset/resource/pdf_file/5/Social_Connectedness_and_Health.pdf

5 Do Pets Improve Health or Life Expectancy?, News Medical http://www.news-medical.net/news/20110804/Do-pets-improve-health-or-life-expectancy.aspx

Simple Health Habit #44 - Practise the Art of Letting Go

1 Barry, M. The Forgiveness Project: The Startling Discovery of How to Overcome Cancer, Find Health, and Achieve Peace. Kregel Publications. 2010. Grand Rapids, Missouri.

2 American Psychological Association. 2006. Forgiveness: A Sampling of Research Results. http://www.apa.org/international/resources/forgiveness.pdf (accessed Dec 2014)

Simple Health Habit #45 - Laugh More

1 University of Maryland Medical Center. Laughter is the "Best Medicine" for Your Heart. http://www.umm.edu/features/laughter.htm#ixzz2OWbc243z

2 University of California. Humor Research Task Force. http://www.ucla.edu/

3 USA Today. Study Links Sense of Humor. http://usatoday30.usatoday.com/tech/science/discoveries/2007-03-13-humor-study_N.htm

4 University of California. Encouraging Your Child's Sense of Humour. http://kidshealth.uclahealth.org/PageManager.jsp?dn=UCLA_Health&lic=311&cat_id=163&article_set=46002&tracking=P_RelatedArticle

5 Don Colbert. The Seven Pillars of Health. 2007, Siloam Publishing, USA.

Simple Health Habit #46 - Recognise Allergies

1 Australasian Society of Clinical Immunology and Allergy. 2010. What is An Allergy. http://www.allergy.org.au/patients/about-allergy/what-is-allergy. (accessed Jan 2015).

Simple Health Habit #47 - Get Some Sunshine

1 Mercola. 2012. Sun Exposure: Benefits Beyond Vitamin D Exposure. http://articles.mercola.com/sites/articles/archive/2012/09/29/sun-exposure-vitamin-d-production-benefits.aspx (accessed Aug 2014).

2 Osteoporosis Australia. 2014. Vitamin D. http://www.osteoporosis.org.au/vitamin-d (accessed Jan 2015).

3 Better Health Channel. 2012. Vitamin D. http://www.betterhealth.vic.gov.au/bhcv2/bhcarticles.nsf/pages/Vitamin_D?open (accessed Jan 2015).

4 Cancer Council Australia. 2014. Sunsmart. http://www.cancer.org.au/preventing-cancer/sun-protection/sunsmart-position-statements.html (accessed Jan 2015).

5 Samanek, A. et al. Estimates of beneficial and harmful sun exposure times during the year for major Australian population centres. Med J Aust 2006; 184 (7): 338-341.

6 Environmental Working Group. 2015. http://www.ewg.org/2014sunscreen/best-sunscreens/best-beach-sport-sunscreens/ (accessed Jan 2015).

7 Australian Prescriber. 2010. Vitamin D Deficiency in Adults. http://www.australianprescriber.com/magazine/33/4/103/6 (accessed Jan 2015).

Simple Health Habit #49 - Ward Off Cancer Cells

1 AIHW. 2008. Cancer. http://www.aihw.gov.au/cancer/ (accessed Jan 2015).

2 Willett, W.C. Diet, nutrition and avoidable cancer. Environ Health Perspect. 1995; 103:175-70.

3 Schatzkin, A. et. Al. 2007. Dietary fiber and whole-grain consumption in relation to colorectal cancer in the NIH-AARP Diet and Health Study. Am J Clin Nutr May 2007 vol. 85 no. 5 1353-1360.

4 Aggarwal, B.B. et al. 2003. Anticancer potential of curcumin: preclinical and clinical studies. Anticancer Res. 2003; 23:363-98.

5 Kotsirilos, V. A Guide to Evidence-Based Integrative and Complementary Medicine. 2011. Elsevier, New South Wales.

6 Colbert, D. Eat This and Live. 2009. Siloam, Florida.

7 Young, C. 2009. Solar ultraviolet radiation and skin cancer. Occup Med (Lond), 59 (2): 82-88.

8 Lavelle, P. 2006. ABC Health and Wellbeing: Is Teflon Safe? http://www.abc.net.au/health/thepulse/stories/2006/02/23/1576391.htm (accessed Jan 2015).

9 Lang, I, Galloway T, Scarlett, A. Association of urinary bisphenol A concentration with medical disorders and laboratory abnormalities in adults. JAMA. 2008; 300:1303-10.

10 Kachhap, S. et al. Cigarette Smoke and Cancer. Journal of Oncology Volume 2011 (2011), Article ID 172678, 2 pages.

11 Thune, I, and Furberg, A. Physical activity in cancer risk: dose-response and cancer, all sites and site-specific. Med Sci Sports Exercise 2001; 33:530-50.

Simple Health Habit #50 - Choose Supplements Wisely

1 Colbert, D. M.D. The Seven Pillars of Health. 2007. Siloam Publishing, USA.

Simple Health Habit #51 - Break Addictions

1 Australian Institute of Professional Counsellors. 2013. Addiction: the biggest killer. http://www.aipc.net.au/articles/addiction-the-biggest-killer/ (accessed Jan 2015).

Simple Health Habit #52 - Cut Yourself Some Slack

1 Neff, Kristin. 2013. Tedx: The Space Between Self-Esteem and Self-Compassion. http://tedxtalks.ted.com/video/The-Space-Between-Self-Esteem-a (accessed Dec 2014).

2 Self-Compassion. Self-Compassion Exercise. http://www.self-compassion.org/self_compassion_exercise.pdf (accessed Dec 2014).

acknowledgements

First and foremost in giving me the encouragement, support, and motivation that I needed to write this book I thank my best friend, and amazing husband, Brad Beer. Your zest for life and endless energy keep life exciting and always moving forward.

To my precious miracle daughter Isabella, thank you for inspiring me to want to be the best role model that I can be as a woman in today's World.

To my overwhelmingly supportive family. You have always believed in me even at times when belief in myself was fading. Your unconditional love has paved the way to express my passion for health without fear of reproach.

Thank you to my publishers Lisa Hanrahan and Paul Dennett from Rockpool Publishing for believing in my dream; including but extending well beyond this book. Thanks too to Katie Evans for doing a fantastic job editing this book with such grace and encouragement.

Lastly I thank my Dad in Heaven, you have loved me from afar yet have been closer than the air I breathe. Thank you for sustaining my heart and soul.

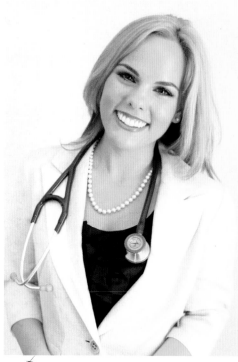

D 60. A.B.

about
Dr Cris Beer

**BBioMedSci, MBBS (hons), FRACGP,
member ACNEM, member AIMA,
Cert IV in Fitness**

As an expert in nutritional medicine Dr Cris specialises not just in the prevention and treatment of illnesses, but in the attaining of optimum health. By employing simple lifestyle and holistic medicine strategies, Dr Cris believes that restoration of health and vitality can be achieved by anyone. Dr Cris holds qualifications in medicine, biomedical science, integrative and nutritional medicine, health coaching, as well as personal fitness training. She was the health consultant for The Biggest Loser Retreat and is sought by the media for regular commentary on radio, TV, newspaper columns, as well as print magazines. She currently practises at The Medical Sanctuary on the Gold Coast as a registered medical doctor helping patients every day. For more information go to drcris.com.au